# THE ESSENTIAL GLUTEN-FREE GUIDE
## How to Go Gluten Free,
## STAY Gluten Free
## and Feel Great!

By Gina M. Williams
Certified Health Coach

The Essential Gluten-Free Guide: How to Go Gluten Free, Stay Gluten Free and Feel Great!

First Printing 2016

ISBN: 978-1537578811

# TABLE OF CONTENTS

Visit us online at: www.healthyana.net

Now you have access to:
- Health tips on how to feed your family better.
- Valuable insights on the truth behind current diet trends.
- Great recipes the whole family will love!

# PREFACE

I am a mom with an analytical mind and a passion for improving my own and my family's health. Another passion of mine is sharing what I have learned on my path to ease the journey of others. These two passions are what led me to become a Certified Health Coach and ultimately what brings us here today.

I knew for years that I needed to cut out gluten, but I kept cheating here and there and fighting with myself about it over and over. I am happy to say that I am FINALLY truly gluten free--no more cheating and I feel amazing!!

Honestly, I feel like a different person! I have more energy, I have lost weight, I am completely rid of the yeast (candida) issues that had plagued my life for over five years. Looking back, none of the cheating was ever "worth it". And I have discovered how to make the change so that I never feel like I am depriving myself. I want you to feel this good too.

This book was born of a deep desire to share with you what I have learned on our family's journey to becoming gluten free, and ultimately much happier and healthier. I do truly hope these lessons and realizations that took me so long to discover will make your journey to living a gluten-free life a success.

With this book you will learn from my many experiences and be empowered with a plan to feel better, lose weight and be a healthier, happier you--all without feeling like you are sacrificing anything...seriously!

# ACKNOWLEDGEMENTS

This book would not have been possible without the unwavering belief and unending love and support of my husband and best friend, Tobin Williams.

Words cannot express my gratitude to Michelle Mueller, Michael Gault, Debby deGennaro, Maura Higgins and Sophia Tracht for helping me untangle my web of words into the book you see today.

# DISCLAIMER

# INTRODUCTION

In this book, you will learn everything you need to know to make your transition to a gluten-free life: easier, tastier, more satisfying, and ultimately successful!

You will learn not only how to find and avoid gluten, but also many powerful and proven methods to a successful gluten-free life, including:

- How to stop feeling like a victim of your gluten intolerance.
- How to create simple meal plans so you don't get stuck without easy gluten-free options.
- How to find gluten-free foods you'll love and that will leave you feeling satisfied.
- How and when to convert your favorite recipes to gluten free.
- How to set yourself up for success with great gluten-free snacks and meals.
- How to use psychology to feel happier about your gluten-free diet and becoming a healthier you.

Plus, you'll get the absolutely essential baking recipes for going gluten free--think bread that tastes like and is the texture of real bread!! You will find over 35 gluten-free recipes that are so good the whole family will love them!

Ultimately, this book is dedicated to giving you all of the tools you need to successfully become gluten free and feeling great!

# CHAPTER 1

## THIS BOOK IS FOR YOU IF YOU...

Each section of this book is designed to walk you through the transition to eating gluten free. But first, is it the right fit for you? How will you benefit in your unique situation? Well, let's take a look...

## Are You Just Starting Out

If you are just starting out you will learn step by step how to transition to a gluten-free diet. You will learn how to spot gluten-containing ingredients, how to make a list of gluten-free foods you already love and also the key substitutions to make your gluten-free transition a success!

## Want to Stop Cheating

Have you been trying to eat gluten free, but you can't seem to stop accidentally, or not so accidentally, eating gluten?

If you are having trouble staying gluten free you will learn how to set yourself up for success by making sure you have easy gluten-free options when you need them.

## Want to Feel Empowered

Do you find yourself being grumpy or even whiny about your gluten-free diet? Do you sometimes feel like a victim of your gluten-free life? If you do, you're not alone.

Here you will learn how to use psychology to change your way of thinking. You will be empowered to transition to a healthier you.

## Want Tastier Options

Are you tired of bread that looks and tastes like cardboard and pasta that's more like paste than something you should eat?

Would you love to know which brands have the best gluten-free bread, pasta, flour and more? If so, you'll find that too.

## Want To Cook For Others

Perhaps you have a loved one who is gluten free and you'd like to be able to help him or her or to know how to prepare a gluten-free meal so that he or she feels included. You will learn not only how to spot gluten-containing ingredients on packaging, but also which substitutions you can use to make your favorite family dishes gluten free. And you'll also find over 35 tested and approved gluten-free recipes!

## Aren't Sure

Are you wondering if cutting out gluten is right for you? These days you hear so much about it, but how can you be sure? Is gluten really bad for you? Is it bad for everyone? Yep, we talk about that as well.

In fact, let's start there…

## Gluten - Real Issue or Trendy Scapegoat?

Simply put, gluten is a protein found in cereal grains such as wheat, barley, rye and other related grains. This gluten protein is found within the grain kernel or seed and it gives wheat flour its elastic properties that make baked goods so deliciously airy and chewy.

So if gluten is just a protein, why is it so bad? Well, it's not inherently bad. This fact raises skepticism about the benefits that thousands of people have reported seeing as a direct result of cutting gluten out of their diets.

Also, the gluten-free industry is growing like gangbusters and many people wonder why? Is it just another diet trend that food producers are capitalizing on and we are just buying into it? Is it all based on hype and claims of weight loss and increased energy? Or do we have a real problem growing in our guts?

All this skepticism makes gluten the topic of much debate and speculation. Here is what we do know:

It is obvious that for the many with celiac disease gluten is a real problem. Those with an allergy to wheat and other non-celiac gluten intolerances must also avoid gluten to avoid serious consequences.

...but what about everyone else?

For more information on the basics of gluten and its related diseases, intolerances and sensitivities see Appendix A.

Certainly, part of this quick growth (maybe even the majority of it) is due to uninformed consumers just hoping for a way to shed a few pounds. But how many of these people opting for gluten-free alternatives are finding that they do indeed feel better? Perhaps they have reduced joint pain, and have less gas, bloating and other intestinal issues. Maybe they even find that on a gluten-free diet they seem to have less brain fog or their children have more control over their emotions and fewer tantrums. And if they do see these types of changes will they stick with it? Only time will tell.

Instead of asking, *Is this a fad?* the more interesting question might be, *why are these issues and allergies all of a sudden such a big part of our lives and is gluten itself really the culprit?* Fifteen years ago--heck, maybe even five years ago--most of us had never even heard of gluten. What happened? People often assume that it's just increased diagnosis and/or awareness, but if you look at the bigger picture of how our diets have changed over the last 60 years, it paints an interesting picture.

For instance, how has wheat changed over the last 60 years? Beginning in the 1950's and continuing in the 1990's wheat in the United States has been hybridized using new methods to increase yield and create a tougher, pest-resistant plant. The industry also wanted a wheat with a longer shelf life. This hybridization over many decades has changed our wheat dramatically.

## Hybridization vs. Genetic Modification

Hybridization should not be confused with genetic modification. Hybridization is a form of gene selection that has been used in agriculture for centuries. In the most basic terms, when hybridizing plants the grower only allows plants with desired characteristics to remain in the gene pool of their gardens or farms. This results in a higher probability that those characteristics, such as watermelons with fewer seeds and sweeter flesh, will be present in their crop.

Genetic modification, on the other hand, is a process which involves the insertion of genes from an entirely different species, such as a virus or bacteria, into the DNA of a plant or animal to insert desired characteristics into the

the species. Some such characteristics in crops that have been genetically modified and are prevalent in our food here in the United States are resistance to weed killers or production of pesticides within the plants themselves. When it comes to genetic modification, we do not know the extent to which humans or their gut bacteria will be altered by this process.

Currently there are a number of a genetically modified organisms (GMOs) that are being grown and consumed every day in this country including: corn, soy, canola, sugar beets, and cotton to name a few. A GMO wheat is being tested, but it has not, at the time of this writing, been approved for commercial production.[5]

The growing and harvesting of wheat itself has changed as well. A recent development, for instance, is an application of the weed killer or herbicide, Round-up®, about a week prior to harvest.[1] This is done to speed up the drying process and some say to increase yields.[2] I can't tell you what percentage of wheat crops are subject to this practice, as estimates vary greatly ranging from 5-80% depending on the region, wheat variety and the source of the information.[3] I can tell you that the fact that any percentage of conventionally grown wheat is subjected to this practice is alarming.

Now, just for fun, consider the fact that for thousands of years our bodies have come to expect varied diets consisting of whole foods that change seasonally. With the incremental addition of store-bought processed foods that are produced using increasing amounts of fillers (namely: wheat, corn, soy and sugar) our diets are no longer varied at all. As you walk down the supermarket aisles, you are presented with what looks like more options and variety than could be imagined... yet when it gets right down to it, it's all made from the same ultra-processed ingredients. Wheat, along with corn, sugar and soy, is present in a wide variety of products where you would never expect them to be. As a result, our bodies are beginning to react like they are under attack. Food allergies alone have increased by over 400% in the last 20 years.[4] Is this due to the lack of variety in our diets, the processing of our foods or something else entirely? No one knows, but it's about time we start asking the question and looking for answers.

So, is gluten free a fad or our future? That I cannot tell you, but what I do know is what I've seen for myself--more and more people finding increased health and vitality when they remove gluten from their diets. Whether it is the gluten itself, the modern wheat that we have cultivated, the overuse of chemical pesticides and herbicides or even the overuse of wheat itself in our processed foods, we may never know. But does it really matter? If you feel better when you cut something out of your diet--you feel better. Isn't that what's most important?

Should everyone go gluten free? No, I don't believe that everyone would benefit from removing gluten from their diets. I do, however, think that organic wheat, which is grownwithout the use of chemically derived pesticides or herbicides, should be strongly considered for anyone who chooses not to go gluten free and has the means to buy organic.

For more information on Roundup® and how it affects our bodies see Appendix B.

# CHAPTER 2

## THE GLUTEN-FREE MIND

Change Your Mind, Change Your Journey

Going gluten free is a journey. It is important to remind ourselves of that because all too often we are pushed or push ourselves to make extreme changes to our lives and routines, but we're only human. We are creatures of habit and extremes are not often sustainable. Lasting change comes by first changing your mindset and then making small sustainable changes in the right direction.

Going gluten free is a journey for all of us, especially those who must cut out gluten immediately and completely, such as is the case for those with celiac disease. It is a journey from eating "normally" to arriving at the point where you are eating gluten free and it feels normal. It can happen and I am going to help you get there. You can do this!!

## The First Step to Going Gluten Free

If you are like many people when you started to go gluten free in the past you began, understandably, by cutting things out of your diet. And for many, like myself, that is all you did to transition. If this describes you, there is a good chance you either fell back into cheating occasionally, eating gluten all the time, or you felt deprived and grumpy about what you couldn't eat--or all of the above. The trouble is when you just jump right into cutting things out you miss the first step to making a real lasting dietary change.

Making changes to our diets, in any way, is something that we all struggle with--just look at how many books, blogs and magazine covers talk about it. But why? Sure, part of it is that food and eating is closely connected to our habits and of course we are evolutionarily programmed to crave calorie dense foods, but more than that, our struggles are rooted in the fact that food is so closely associated with family, love, warmth and security.

These connections mean that making changes to our diets can be very emotionally charged. For this very reason, the first step must be to take a look at our mindset and our thoughts on the subject. Are you feeling sad, grumpy or victimized by these changes? Or do you feel in control, confident and empowered to better your health? This initial perspective can make all the difference in your success, which is why the first step to going gluten free must be to look at your mindset.

The good news is changing your diet doesn't have to make you grumpy or land you on an emotional roller coaster. Avoiding the drama is simple, but will take a bit of prep work. I promise it won't take long and it will be well worth it.

## Making The Journey Easier

In order to successfully change the way you eat, that is without cheating and without feeling cheated, you must change your mindset. If you are going to make a real lasting change you must figure out a way to get those whiny voices in your head on board--or at the very least have a great comeback for them when they try to argue with you.

It's just three simple steps, but these three steps will make all the difference in making your journey to being gluten free, happier, healthier and more successful!

These 3 steps will guide you to do just that:

1.  You need an excellent *why*--a reason that resonates deeply with you. We will talk more about finding your *why* in a bit.

2.  You must have a definitive goal and time frame set before you begin. Are you looking to cut out gluten for the long haul or just experimenting to find out if gluten really is a problem for you? It makes a difference and I'll explain why.

3.  You must believe in your goal to your core. Whether your goal is to cure your leaky gut or just to see how you feel without gluten in your diet you must believe in your goal to be successful.

If you are thinking that this sounds too obvious, like an unnecessary step or even a waste of time, I assure you it is not. Let me tell you why. Finding and putting into real terms the answers to these questions will give you the "willpower" it takes to stick with it. Going gluten free is not something you go half way on if you want to see and feel results. You really must stick to it--100%, no cheating. We'll talk more about why in Chapter 3, but what you need to take away here is that these three steps are the key not only to sticking with it, but also to feeling good about your decision.

You may have noticed that the word "willpower" above is in quotations... that was no accident. This journey of mine that spans over 10 years has led me to the conclusion that there is no such thing as willpower, at least not in the way people talk about it. *Man, George, you sure do have a lot of willpower.* If willpower existed in this way then some people, those who are blessed with it, would always do exactly what they set out to do and would never struggle to complete a goal or perform a necessary duty. Those without willpower would flail about constantly failing to accomplish anything at all.

If willpower was something that you cultivated, practiced and maintained it would be consistent across all parts of your life. You would have the same amount of willpower to get up or leave the house on time as you would to stick to your budget each month. But that isn't what we see in life. We are surrounded by people of all levels and classes who excel and are motivated to go above and beyond when it comes to some things and yet fight themselves daily and fail miserably over and over again when it comes to other things. So, what is it that sets certain actions up for success while others are destined for failure?

In short, it's passion. It's the artist who will do anything for his art--go without sleep, forego food, perform physical feats and maintain a brutal schedule, but when it's not about art he struggles to follow through. He tries to plan and make progress, but fails to deliver and disappoints himself over and over. It's belief. Take me for example. I have always struggled to stick to a routine. I don't do anything with any regularity and I have never been able to take daily vitamins more than once a week...maybe. But when I was pregnant I took those vitamins every day religiously. Why? Because I had a clear, concise, very specific reason to take them and I believed to my core. I wanted the very best for my baby and it was my belief that this vitamin was essential to giving my child the best start possible.

If you look, I'll bet you will find that you too have great "willpower" when it comes to some things, and that you constantly struggle when it comes to other things. Since willpower doesn't exist, at least not in the traditional sense, you or anyone can find the will simply by going through these three steps. I believe you'll find, as I have, that when you have the *will* the *power* just comes.

Let's dig a little deeper into the three steps. Then you can take just a few minutes to really think them through and you will be on your way to a successful, happy, healthy, gluten-free life.

## Step #1: Your Deepest Why

To change your diet, or any part of your lifestyle or habits you need an excellent reason--an answer to the question *why?*. Why ask why? Because you will need it to stay strong. You will need it to have the willpower, the resolve, not to have a bite of that doughnut or just one little Christmas cookie. You will also need it so that you don't waiver when the gremlin in your head or the guy in the next cubicle questions your decision to go gluten free.

And you don't just need any *why* if you are going to stick with it to see the amazing results, you are going to need your *why* and it has to resonate deeply with you.

So ask yourself, "Why do I want to go gluten free?". You could say, "I want to feel better", "I want to lose weight" or "I want to stop feeling sick"; and while those do answer the question, they aren't enough. Those answers are the equivalent of saying, "fine" when an acquaintance asks how you are doing. We all say, "fine" no matter how we are really doing--there is no depth there. The kind of *why* we are looking for to motivate you and help you on your gluten-free journey is deeper and more personal--something you might only tell a close friend or even something you might consider completely private.

Look at these four statements and notice how they resonate differently:

- I want to manage my Hashimoto's so that I have energy to play with my children. (Ok...)
- I want to reduce my joint pain so I can go golfing. (Sure...)
- I want to feel good enough to have great sex again. (Now we are talking!)
- I want to cure my leaky gut or my eczema because I want to feel sexy and confident like I did years ago. (Yes!)

Can you see how these different statements have different feelings behind them? While wanting to feel better and have more energy to play with your children is a great goal, you must ask yourself if it's really enough to motivate you.

For instance, wanting to be around to meet your grandkids is a fine and noble *why*, but we are creatures looking for immediate gratification. Which do you think will win--the doughnut right in front of you or the grandkids you don't have yet? Yep, that's what used to happen to me. And that is why finding and defining your deepest *why*--the one that really touches your soul--makes such a difference!

Also, it really helps to make your *why* feel real and attainable if there is some immediacy to it. If you can create a sense of urgency within yourself it will be an even better motivator.

Here are some examples of a *why* that creates a sense of urgency:

- I want to have energy to play with my kids <u>this summer</u>.
- I want to feel good enough to go golfing in 3 or 6 months and <u>plan a trip so you have a timeframe</u>.
- I want to heal my irritable bowel and lose this bloating because I want to feel sexy and confident for my <u>anniversary or high school reunion (something with a specific date)</u>.
- I want to clear up my rosacea so that I feel beautiful again <u>before the holidays</u>--yep, I said it. It can be done and for me cutting out gluten was the first step to clearing up my rosacea.

Adding that timeline to your reason for going gluten free not only creates a sense of urgency, but it re-categorizes the whole idea in your mind. Now, it's a priority. Now, this image of a better you is right there in front of you; it's real.

For some, the answer to the question "*Why?*" will come easily. If you are feeling really sick and you know that cutting out gluten works to take away your symptoms it's simple--you want to feel better. But even in this example drilling down is still important. Let me explain.

Let's say, you've been feeling so very ill and you recently, or not so recently, found that cutting gluten out of your diet helps tremendously. First, I am sorry that you have to deal with this and that you have been feeling so sick. I am also thankful that you have found something that gives you some relief. I understand that for you, your *why* seems so obvious, but just because you feel better physically doesn't mean that it will be easy emotionally.

Getting deeper into answering your *why* question will help you to see the light at the end of the tunnel and to focus on the positive outcome. When you do, it works wonders to make you feel good about your goal. When you dig deeper it makes going gluten free *your* decision, *your* outcome--as opposed to feeling like a victim of your situation--deflated or even depressed. When you feel like improving your health is *your* decision you begin to feel empowered, stronger and more confident. It can make a world of difference in how you feel, the success of your gluten-free journey and above all your improved quality of life and health!

So, how do you find your deepest *why?* Try this exercise--ask yourself "why?" five or even ten times each time digging deeper. It might go something like this:

1. *Why* do I want to go gluten free? Because I want to feel better.
2. *Why* do I want to feel better? Because I want to have more energy.
3. *Why* do I want to have more energy? Because I want to get out there and do what I love.

And keep going, trying to get more and more specific and more and more positive with each answer. Then use those answers to build a very specific *why* that resonates deeply with you.

No one needs to see your answers. They are personal and private to you so be honest, be true to yourself and you will find your deepest *why*.

You may find that you need to go through this exercise more than once. For some people the first time you go through it, your answers may be negatively charged, and that is okay. Just let the answers come. Sometimes you need to get that negativity out. If you find this to be true for you, when you are done the first time just step away for a bit, get some water or take a quick walk and then come back to it and start over on a fresh sheet of paper. This time try to ask the questions with a smile. I know it sounds a little nuts, but it will help put you in a positive place.

And remember, it doesn't matter if you do the exercise once or ten times, you will know when you have gotten the answers you can work with. You should be looking to build a statement that leaves you emotionally charged and excited. When you find that you'll know you have found the *why* that will help you succeed. And it will change your journey.

As you go through this exercise be sure that you don't get caught up in the "How?". Your answers shouldn't go into *how* you will achieve the outcome you are looking for, but should focus only on what you want your outcome to be. Define what is missing from your life and how going gluten free can improve it.

This first step was the tough one. Now that you have your deepest why the next steps are a snap!

## Step #2: Define Your Immediate Goal and Timeline

Now that you have this vision on where you want to be (and hopefully a timeframe of when you'd like to get there), you need a plan on how to get there. You need to define an immediate attainable goal with a timeline.

After years of battling with myself over gluten, trying and failing, cheating and feeling cheated, I finally got to the point where I found my deepest *why*. I knew what I wanted and I wasn't even sure that cutting out gluten would get me there, but I knew I wanted to give it a real chance. I wanted to find out once and for all how much of a difference it would make to cut gluten entirely out of my diet.

So, I started with just 21 days--21 days <u>completely</u> gluten free. Three weeks is the <u>minimum</u> amount of time it takes to begin to see the benefits of a gluten-free diet. At the end of that 21 days my plan was to reassess--was I convinced one way or the other or did I need to extend the time?

Having a definite timeframe made such a difference for me. It was long enough (just barely) to test and see if it would make me feel better. And it was short enough that I felt I could make it.

This made sense to me. For you it might be a week, a month or six months. Whatever it is, setting a specific goal with a timeframe is important because you create a certain expectation for yourself. When you attempt to make a change to your diet, or any other part of your life for that matter; you must have a specific timeframe or you will make it easy for yourself to postpone indefinitely or give up completely.

Remember, this is a journey. So if your journey begins with just a week that's fine. You'll need to keep in mind that that a week isn't long enough to see all the benefits of going gluten free. But by completing a goal of any length--a week or even a day, you can experience all of the good things that come from finishing something you start. That boost of self-confidence, pride of completion and knowing that you can do it!

Putting your goal into a timeframe also gives you a defined endpoint. Something to stop the excuses and procrastination. You can also see that even if your goal is only a day or a week, you will still enjoy the benefits of making it through and feeling the can-do spirit that will help you set bigger goals for yourself. Put that energy and positivity to work and make a new goal right away. Build on that momentum.

Sometimes, all you need is a few quick wins to give you the confidence to get to where you want to be.

## Step #3:  Believe It To Your Core

Your goal must be something you want deeply and believe at your core. If you have doubts that gluten is really a problem for you, don't just keep beating your head against the wall and fighting with yourself. Instead, do a little research. Read up on your symptoms and find out what other people have found when they cut out gluten. There will always be people who don't believe it works. All that matters for this exercise is what <u>you</u> believe.

The very fact that you are reading this book means that you already believe going gluten free may help you feel better and improve your health. And that may be all you need to try eliminating gluten completely for 21 days. As I mentioned in step two, this is the very minimum amount of time it takes to *begin* to see what effect it has on your body. For me it was obvious.

When I finally went completely gluten free after years of trying, cheating, and failing miserably, I saw how great I could and should be feeling--and there was no turning back. You may or may not have the same result, but when you believe your effort is worth it (even if it's only that you want to give going gluten free a fair try)--it makes all the difference. Then you can commit and find your will.

For more information on research studies and other resources on gluten-related symptoms see the resource section in Chapter 10.

And believing that gluten is a possible source for your suffering isn't the only thing you must believe in. You also have to believe in your goal. Is it realistic for you? Do you think you can do it? It is best to choose a goal that is just slightly out of your comfort zone, that is believable, but will also push you just a tad. Belief is crucial. Will only works if you believe in your goal.

So to recap, changing your mind will change your journey. It will make going gluten free *your* choice and will bring what you desire. And it's as simple as following these three steps:

1. You need to find your *why*--your deep, personal desire that gives you an emotionally charged reason for going gluten free.
2. You need to define your goal and your timeframe. How long are you going to go gluten free and at what point do you want to celebrate your progress and reassess.
3. You need to be sure you truly believe in your goal.

These three steps will set you on a path to a happier, healthier, gluten-free life. Your transition to a gluten-free life will still be a process, and truly that's okay, but it doesn't have to be a battle.

# CHAPTER 3

## HOW TO AVOID GLUTEN

B efore we dig into the specific steps that will guide you to what you can eat in your new gluten-free life we need to go over a few basics when it comes to avoiding gluten.

When beginning a gluten-free diet you might expect that you simply need to remove breads, cookies, crackers and other baked goods made from wheat flour, right?

Unfortunately, it's just not that clear cut. In this chapter we will discuss gluten (and non-gluten) containing grains, hidden sources of gluten and we'll even touch on cross-contamination.

## Where Gluten is Found

In Chapter 1 we discussed that gluten is a protein found in certain cereal grains. The most common of the gluten-containing grains is wheat. So, people often assume if something is wheat-free that it's also gluten free. That is not necessarily the case.

Gluten is found in a number of cereal grains. So, exactly which grains contain gluten? Here is a list of common grains to avoid:

- Wheat
- Barley
- Rye
- Spelt
- Graham

- Durham
- Bulgar
- Faro
- Kamut®
- Semolina

So which grains don't contain gluten? The following common grains and flours are suitable for a gluten-free diet:

- All nuts
- All seeds
- All beans
- All varieties of rice
- Oats
- Quinoa
- Sorghum
- Tapioca
- Amaranth
- Millet
- Buckwheat--Yes… buckwheat.

Now, there is something you must know about these gluten-free grains. **They are truly gluten free only if they are labeled gluten free and processed in a gluten-free facility (which should be the case if they are labeled gluten free).** If they are not labeled gluten free, chances are they were processed in a shared facility along with gluten-containing grains and do have at least trace amounts of gluten. We will talk more about this in the cross-contamination section later.

The good news is, with the gluten-free market growing so quickly, most of these grains are widely available and many of them will be labeled gluten free.

So, now that we know what grains to look for to avoid gluten and which grains and flours are gluten free we have a good start. The next step to avoiding gluten is understanding the hidden sources of gluten.

## Names Can Fool You

For instance, buckwheat has the word wheat right in the name, but in fact is another plant species entirely. Buckwheat is not a true cereal grain and contains no gluten.

However, buckwheat pancakes at a conventional (not gluten free) restaurant contain regular wheat flour as well as buckwheat flour and are not gluten free. Same goes for soba noodles which are made from a combination of buckwheat and wheat flour.

What about cornbread? Sounds safe, right? But again, unless it is specifically made to be gluten free, it contains wheat flour.

# How to Spot Hidden Sources of Gluten

In order to remove gluten from your diet you need to understand that gluten is not only found in the obvious places like baked goods, but it is also in many less obvious places such as croutons, fried chicken, gravy, meatloaf and even beer to name a few. Plus, it's also used as a thickener and/or filler in all kinds of processed foods. Let's begin by looking at some foods that you might think are gluten free, but that actually are not. Cornbread, for instance, seems like it would be safe, but cornbread often contains regular flour as well as cornmeal. So, unless it specifically says it is gluten free, it probably isn't.

Here's a list of some of the gluten-containing foods that are most commonly mistaken as gluten free:

- Couscous
- Gnocchi
- Soba noodles
- Chow mein
- Cornbread
- Potato bread
- Graham crackers
- Granola
- Panko breadcrumbs
- Tabbouleh
- Gravy

- Soy sauce
- Cheesecake
- Some tortilla chips (made from flour tortillas)

The good news is that these ingredients will have the word wheat under the ingredients section of the label. And it will also read in bold print, "CONTAINS: WHEAT" which makes it really easy to double check if you aren't sure. Although that is not the only source of gluten, it is the most common and will help you easily rule out products that contain wheat.

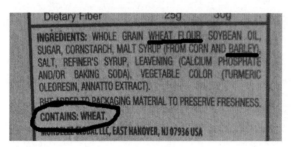

Look for this on the ingredients label.

If you see this on the label you can be sure that the food in question contains gluten. If you don't see it, that doesn't mean it is gluten free. You will need to investigate further, looking for other sources of gluten before deciding if it is indeed gluten free.

For anyone that needs to cut out all gluten here is a list of ingredients that do contain gluten unless specifically labeled as gluten free:

- Malt (including malt vinegar and malt seasoning)
- Caramel coloring
- Caramel flavor
- Soy sauce
- Brown rice syrup
- Seitan (used in vegetarian mock meats)
- Brewers yeast
- Liquid smoke (anything barbeque flavored)

I know this seems to be getting very complicated, but there is an easier solution for store bought foods. **The best way to ensure that the products you buy are gluten free is to purchase items specifically labeled gluten free.**

The FDA does not regulate where or how companies label their products, but they do regulate the meaning behind these four terms[6]:

- "Gluten-free"
- "Free of gluten"
- "No gluten"
- "Without gluten"

By law these terms on a food label are required to have a gluten content of less than 20 parts per million (ppm), an amount low enough that is tolerated well by most gluten-intolerant individuals as stated by the FDA.[7]

This makes eating gluten free at home much easier, but it becomes trickier when eating out. There are some truly hidden forms of gluten that you may not realize are in prepared foods. To be on the safe side here is a list of foods you should avoid when eating out:

- Lunch meat
- Cheap ground beef
- Hamburgers with fillers
- Hot dogs
- Marinades
- French fries
- Hashbrowns
- Soups
- Broths
- Salad dressing

These lists are a good start to identifying some of the most common sources of hidden gluten. If you are particularly sensitive you should really click your way over to: www. celiac.org/live-gluten-free/glutenfreediet/ to learn all about the possible sources of gluten including less common food additives, supplements, medicines and other non-food sources of gluten.

For a printable list of gluten-free grains and flours as well as which foods to avoid, visit: www.healthyana.net/essentialgf

## Cross-Contamination

Cross-contamination is a real problem for many people afflicted with celiac disease, wheat allergy or other major gluten intolerances. For some, being in the same room with airborne wheat can result in a reaction[8], for others even direct contamination, a shared toaster, cutting board or condiment utensil is not an issue at all. You must consider your own personal sensitivity level to gluten to decide if it will be a problem for you.

When it comes to cross-contamination, here is what you need to know:

- Wheat flour can remain airborne for hours. So, anything made in any kitchen, bakery or food processing plant that is not a dedicated gluten-free facility is, at least to some degree, contaminated with gluten.
- Oils used for deep frying will contain gluten if the restaurant fries anything containing gluten.
- Oats are easily contaminated because they are often processed in facilities that also process wheat products. Gluten-free oats are processed in a gluten-free facility and are considered safe.

With this information and knowing your own individual sensitivity level, you and your doctor can determine where you need to draw the line.

## Who Needs to be Concerned With Hidden Gluten

To answer this question you need to look at your own personal level of gluten sensitivity or intolerance.

I want to be perfectly clear--if your doctor has prescribed a gluten-free diet for you, you must consult with him or her to determine the extent of gluten contamination that will affect you. In many cases, doctors are simply trying to restrict foods that inherently contain gluten from your diet including added flour and thickeners. And that is what I focus on in this book.

If you have severe reactions please be sure to review the resources mentioned in this chapter and those at the end of the book for guidance on how to be watchful of hidden gluten and how to find restaurants that are dedicated gluten free to avoid cross-contamination. You may even consider requesting a referral to a registered dietitian to help you through the process of changing your diet.

If you do not have severe reactions and have not been told by your doctor that you need to be on a strict gluten-free diet that is completely free of gluten contamination, the question of gluten free or gluten light (allowing for some contamination) really comes down to your reason for cutting gluten out.

If you simply want to eat better and maybe shed a few pounds, no problem. Cutting out gluten can guide you toward healthier food options by limiting the amount of processed foods you eat.

However, the growing popularity of the gluten-free diet has come with increased availability of gluten-free junk foods-- snacks, cookies, cakes, pizzas and more. And if losing weight is your goal it is worth noting that gluten-free flour blends often contain more carbohydrates and have a higher glycemic index than wheat flour. So those gluten-free junk foods may be worse for you than the regular wheat options you are trying to avoid. In this scenario, where a person is cutting out gluten just to cut down on carbohydrates, going gluten free versus gluten light is not terribly important and you certainly shouldn't spend any energy worrying about cross-contamination.

I will say, however, that most people I have coached find it is easier to monitor themselves with clearly defined rules. That is to say, they find it easier to cut something out completely than to try to limit themselves. If you are one of those people you may want to go completely gluten free (no cheating) if only to keep one handful of chips or a couple of crackers from turning into a constant battle.

If, on the other hand, you are looking at cutting out gluten because you feel better when you do, or you want to find out if a gluten-free diet will relieve some of your symptoms, then you really should do your best to be gluten free and not just gluten light. You may not need to worry about cross-contamination at a restaurant that isn't a dedicated gluten-free space, but you will benefit most by cutting foods that contain gluten completely out of your diet.

I can tell you from my own experience and the experiences of those that I have helped through the transition that it makes a huge difference! I was at least 90% gluten free for over two years, and though I felt better my symptoms were by no means gone. They would flare up on a pretty regular basis. Now I am talking about just a few bites of a gluten-containing food once a week or a beer here and there. These small cheats kept me from really feeling better and getting the results I was hoping to see.

It wasn't until I decided to really commit to the practice of eating completely gluten free that I experienced how good I could feel. In the beginning I committed to only 21 days--just 3 weeks--to decide if I should stick to this gluten-free lifestyle or if I should stop fighting with myself and abandon it once and for all.

By the end of the third week, it was clear that I felt much better and that the things I had thought were "worth it" when I cheated for those two years were never really worth it. I had symptoms from skin rashes to chronic systemic yeast infections that completely cleared up in those first three weeks.

I felt really good for the first time in years and, as an added bonus, my rosacea improved tremendously. It was too obvious to dismiss, the fact is that gluten was causing me some seriously undue stress and honestly making me feel really crappy.

This makes perfect sense when you think about what non-celiac gluten sensitivity is and how it affects your body. The reaction your body is having appears to be an over-reactive immune response. That immune response isn't going to lessen if you continue to allow the invader, in this case gluten, into your body. Your immune system will remain on high alert until you remove the source of the reaction completely.

There is some (at this point anecdotal) evidence that if we can give our bodies a rest from this bombardment for 6 months to a year and then slowly--very slowly, as in a teaspoon a day and build up from there--reintroduce the offending substance (gluten) that the immune response may lessen or in some cases go away completely. This would allow those with a sensitivity to gluten to once again enjoy foods that contain gluten in moderation. This is a promising theory, but let me be clear--this is NOT in the case of celiac or a true wheat allergy. This MIGHT be a possibility in the case of some food sensitivities. And, of course, you should always consult your doctor.

So, you can see that, for anyone cutting out gluten for medical reasons, going gluten free all the way and cutting it out to the greatest extent possible is absolutely the way to go. If this makes your heart sink a little, have no fear. The next chapter will fix you right up!

## Dealing with Multiple Food Allergies or Intolerances

What if gluten isn't the only thing you are avoiding? Often when it is recommended that you cut gluten out of your diet it is also recommended that you cut out other foods. Those foods are usually one or more of the following: dairy, sugar, soy, corn, eggs and/or caffeine. When you first hear this it can be daunting news--it's a lot to take in. But the good news is you can still use the principles in this book to guide your journey. You will just need to keep your unique situation in mind when you are going through the exercises and building your lists.

## My Personal Elimination Diet

Full disclosure in those first three weeks I cut out not only gluten, but also dairy, corn, eggs, caffeine and alcohol. These were the most likely culprits to be causing symptoms for me personally.

Then I added everything (except gluten) back in, one item every week, so that I could track what gave me issues. In the end, I found that all of my symptoms pointed toward gluten as the culprit. I also found that when I added dairy back in, I developed a new symptom that I had never had before, eczema.

When I realized that the onset of my eczema coincided with the addition of dairy back into my diet, I removed it again and it cleared up immediately. I was amazed!

Many doctors suggest cutting out the following list of common culprits when going through an elimination diet: wheat, gluten, refined sugar, corn, eggs, dairy, and soy.

For more info on elimination diets visit:
www.healthyana.net/ed

# CHAPTER 4

## WHAT CAN I EAT?

The Key to a Successful Gluten-Free Life

Okay, so we have taken a little time to prepare your mind for this transition, and I promise it will be worth it! And now you know how to spot and avoid gluten on ingredient lists. Finally, we've made it to the part you've been waiting for...*Just tell me what I can eat!!*

## The Most Important Part of Changing Your Diet

This is another little tip that I hope will help you immensely. It is so obvious, yet few people see the opportunity. Most people (myself included) when they discover that they should remove gluten from their diet, they do just that--remove it, but they don't change anything else. They keep eating the same way and the same things just replacing the delicious bread or crackers that they love with some sub-par crumbly styrofoam-like alternative.

Long before I was anywhere near a gluten-free path, I struggled for years with infertility. During that time, one of my doctors suggested I try a wheat-free, dairy-free diet to increase my health and hopefully our odds. I was willing to try anything.

I stuck with this elimination diet for the better part of a year, and I didn't cheat once. I told you I would have done anything to get that baby. Truly, looking back it was a miracle that I made it that long. I had done NOTHING to change my eating habits, I had simply removed the stuff I couldn't have and in many instances replaced it with things I hated, like oatmeal, rice bread and corn tortillas.

Now don't get me wrong, these things may have their place, but at this time in my life I was working full time, going to college full time and I was on the run a lot. This meant that I wasn't just eating oatmeal, I was eating cold oatmeal that had more in common with the paste you used in kindergarten than actual food. It's no wonder I didn't get pregnant while on that diet--I was miserable.

This type of food elimination from your diet without finding proper replacements that satisfy you is the first and biggest mistake you can make when trying to change your diet in any way. There are two problems with this approach.

First, when you only remove things from your diet, you focus only on what you can't have and it's very unsatisfying. I know because I've been there, I've walked in those shoes. Everywhere you look you see what you used to eat and everything you can no longer eat. And that makes the transition more difficult than it needs to be.

Second, who wants to eat sub-par alternatives? Food at its core is not just food, it's a sensory experience and we should enjoy it! There is no reason that your gluten-free life should be void of good foods that you love--there is a better way!

So what do you do? You MUST find, and always be on the lookout for, satisfactory replacements if you are going to succeed. And when I say succeed, I don't just mean succeed in eliminating the gluten. I mean reaching toward your goal and feeling good about it. After all, isn't feeling good the point of all this health talk?

If I am gluten free, but grumpy, irritable and bitter that I never get to eat anything good, that's an awful outcome. That can't be considered a success. And honestly, it will never really improve your health. Health involves the body and the mind.

We've already talked a lot about getting your mind on board, but we aren't done yet. Yes, you need your goals to be specific, deep-seated and to make sense to you; but you also need to feel satisfied. That is what we will cover next.

## How to Find Gluten-Free Foods You Will Love

Going gluten free is a journey and you can't start a journey from where you want to be. It all starts from where you are right now. So, how do you find gluten-free foods you will love? You begin with all of the gluten-free foods you already eat and love. I am going to ask you to write a list of all the foods that you love deeply which are inherently gluten free. They don't even have to be good for you, just gluten free.

My list would look like this:

- Great glass of orange juice
- Steamed broccoli with balsamic vinegar

- Crisp apple
- Tomatoes with salt and pepper
- Avocados
- Pesto
- Grilled chicken (brining is a must!)
- Roasted sweet potato or acorn squash
- Beef and bell pepper salad
- Italian potato salad (we use oil/vinegar instead of mayo)
- Grilled corn on the cob
- Build-your-own salad night
- Vegetable soup with rice
- Tomatoes with fresh basil and balsamic vinegar
- Meatball soup (GF meatballs)
- Grilled fish tacos
- Beef tacos
- Fried rice (GF soy sauce)
- Fajita bowls
- Chili
- Corn tortilla chips and salsa or guacamole
- Trail mix
- Kombucha
- Whiskey :)
- Butternut squash soup
- Veggies and hummus
- Kind® bars
- Chocolate

Getting hungry? And that list is even gluten, soy, egg AND dairy free--you get the idea. You can do this! It's an important step to inspiring yourself to think creatively about the things you already love. Then you find a few key substitutions and voilà--you have so many options!!!

Be sure to build the list in a place that's easily accessible: your phone, calendar, on the fridge--whatever is close by. When it's within reach you'll look at often and can add more things as you think of them.

This is exciting stuff!

Go ahead. Put the book down right now and begin building this list. There's no time like the present--I'll wait.

(cue the Jeopardy® music)

Now you have started your list, and hopefully gotten some of your creative juices flowing. Keep adding to that list and building on it as you expand your new food horizons.

## Finding Acceptable Alternatives

Now comes the most important step of building your list-- finding acceptable alternatives that will satisfy you. They are out there, I promise. You may have to think outside the box a little, but this is a key step to living a successful, satisfying gluten-free life.

Bread Alternatives

First things first--you need a good gluten-free bread, at least when you first start out. Most gluten-free breads that are available commercially are dense, dry, unflavorful and expensive. Sounds tasty, right?! Worry not, there are other options--you just have to know where to look. These other options are still significantly more expensive than traditional bread, but honestly, if you let the expense guide you it will likely reduce the amount of bread you are eating, which may not be a bad thing.

Eating bread may not be a problem, but as you take a look at how much you have been consuming you may find, like we did, that there is significant room to incorporate more diversity into your grain intake and whole grains at that. Quinoa, millet, wild rice, brown rice and whole gluten-free oats all have significant health benefits and are a great source of fiber when they aren't refined. And that is the reality of any gluten-free bread that tastes and chews like a good bread should--it is very refined. Potato and tapioca starches are present in significant quantities, neither of which have much if anything to offer in the way of nutrition. This isn't a problem, per se, but something to be aware of.

All that said, I believe that a good gluten-free bread makes the transition to a gluten-free lifestyle much easier. You can find the recipe for our family's favorite hassle-free (read; no kneading) bread in Chapter 7, and a guide to our take on commercially available gluten-free breads in Chapter 8, along with some other easy substitutions for pasta and pizza.

<u>Snack Food Alternatives</u>

After bread, the next important acceptable alternative to have in place is your snack foods. Everyone needs a go-to snack. Mine used to be crackers and cheese with apple slices. Well, gluten-free crackers are even more expensive than regular crackers, which were already a splurge in our house, and I'm off dairy as well so that had to change. After gluten-free crackers I tried Glutino® pretzels, which are amazing and do a great job of satisfying the need to crunch, but again they aren't cheap, especially given how hard it is to stop eating them!

Certainly, we do have gluten-free pretzels, crackers and Garden Veggie Straws® on occasion, but for the most part we have transitioned to these snack foods:

- A piece of fruit
- Hard boiled egg
- Trail mix
- Homemade GF muffins
- Homemade energy bars
- Organic corn tortilla chips and salsa
- Beef jerky
- Turkey and corn(or rice) tortilla rolls

- Raw veggies - carrots, bell peppers, cucumbers, jicama
- Kind® or Larabars® when we are on the go

And don't forget fluids! I drink a ton of water, tea and kombucha now so I snack much less than I used to. Whatever you find works for you be sure that it is easy to grab, and that you portion it out for yourself. Put some crackers, carrot sticks, pretzels, or whatever it is into a bowl instead of sitting down with the whole bag or box.

---

### Snack Bars

Larabars® & KIND® Bars are my favorite on-the-go snacks. They have plenty of flavor options and are made with real food ingredients.

Both companies are gluten free, GMO-free and also have many products that remove other common allergens such as dairy, soy and eggs. As always, read the package labels to be sure they are right for you.

---

## Breakfast Alternatives

Breakfast is another tough one for many people. Cereal or toast are common breakfast foods for which you can easily find gluten-free options that are commercially available, but we often opt for some of the following gluten-free alternatives:

- Overnight Oats
- Simple Granola
- Wild Rice Porridge
- Scones
- Muffins
- Quiche
- Pancakes or Waffles

We do this partially to reduce costs, but also once again to broaden our whole-grain horizons. You will find the recipes for all of these in this book as well. And they are all really quite simple and quick.

## Alternative Treats

Being able to treat yourself now and again is an important part of feeling satisfied. Having some gluten-free treats on hand for when you have an urge so that you don't dive into the gluten-full cookie jar is a really good idea.

It could be as simple as some good quality chocolate, ice cream or smoothie makings in the house. My little trick is to have the ingredients to bake a treat on hand at all times so that I have to want it bad enough to actually bake the cookies. In the end I almost always settle for a cup of tea or a handful of chocolate chips. Just remember, this is your journey and whatever it is that works for you, where you are now, is perfect.

I strongly suggest that whatever you decide, be sure that you have some options available. It will ease your transition considerably. And you might even consider putting a stash in your desk drawer at work for those times when birthday cakes and doughnuts are tempting you to stray.

As I mentioned before, we will cover more alternatives when we look into how to convert your favorite recipes to gluten free in Chapter 8.

For now, take a look at the list you made and take a little time to think through how you can mix and match those items into snacks and meals. Also, make note of what is missing so you can continue to find alternatives you will love!

# CHAPTER 5

## STICKING WITH IT

Setting Yourself up for Success

I n order to set yourself up for success the most important thing is to do everything you can to minimize decision fatigue. This is something that took me years to realize, but lucky for you only weeks to master.

If you are unfamiliar with the term, decision fatigue is what happens when you go to the store at 6:30 pm on a Friday night when you are brain-dead, exhausted and starving. You simply cannot be expected to think or make good decisions at a time like this. Your decision-making mojo is all used up. You are in the midst of decision fatigue and destined to make choices that are quick and easy whether or not they are aligned with your goals.

So, how do you escape this familiar territory? At the risk of sounding like a broken record, let's reiterate.

The first step to avoiding decision fatigue is to remember your deep-seated personal *why*.

Why? you ask. Because then taking a few extra minutes each week to make a plan so that you have the items you need, when you need them, is no big deal. It becomes a priority because it's no longer something someone told you to do or something you feel that you should do. Now, being prepared so that you can meet your goal is something you want to do. Something that is now worth it to you.

# A New Approach to Meal Planning

The second step in avoiding decision fatigue is to create a rhythm that makes planning easy for you. Some people might call this a schedule. I prefer to call it a rhythm because it doesn't need to be rigid. There will be times when it gets off track and that's okay, but we have something to come back to. The best part is once you have been doing it for a while it doesn't feel like work--it just feels right.

For our family it works best to have a weekly rhythm and I plan our meals for the week each Sunday. I also like to call it a rhythm because we don't have the same thing every week, but we have the same type of dish on the same day each week. For instance:

- Monday - rice & veggie
- Tuesday - soup and/or salad
- Wednesday - pizza & fresh veggies
- Thursday - meat dish & salad
- Friday - pasta dish & fresh veggies
- Saturday - free day/leftovers
- Sunday - slow cooker recipes

This makes planning really fast and easy. It only takes a few minutes each Sunday and I don't have to think about it for the whole week!

There is a reason some of our parents had meal plans like these; quite simply so they didn't have to think about it! To avoid decision fatigue, Steve Jobs is said to have gone so far as to only wear black so he didn't have to waste brain power making such trivial decisions as what to wear. A weekly meal rhythm is your black outfit--you don't have to dwell on it because it's already decided.

The best part about incorporating a rhythm with your meal planning is not only how easy it makes things, but how versatile it is. Gone are the days of stroganoff Fridays. You don't have to eat the same things over and over because the categories are so loose!

For example on Mondays the rice and veggie dish could be any of the following:

- Quasi Risotto* - flavor options are numerous
- Fried rice* with stir-fried veggies - all varieties (made with GF soy sauce)
- Burrito Bowl*
- Spanish rice with fajitas
- Stuffed bell peppers*
- Rice pilaf and poached or steamed fish
- Rice and bean salad

*I will share recipes for these dishes in Chapter 9

Also, it doesn't have to be just rice. You can switch it up to be quinoa or millet as well. And all of these grains are so easy to throw in the rice cooker and be done!!

A rhythm like this also makes creating your shopping list much easier. You can go once and be set for real meals all week!

You can create the same type of rhythm for breakfast and even lunch if you find that it helps. We do have a rhythm for breakfast as well, but you can also just keep a few items in the house for breakfast if that works for you.

This is what we usually keep in stock:

- Sprouted grains protein shake powder for me
- Gluten-free granola
- Goat milk kefir or yogurt
- Gluten-free muffin, scone and pancake ingredients
- Almond butter for gluten-free toast
- Gluten-free oatmeal
- And the occasional boxed gluten-free cereal

We also often use leftover rice or millet from dinners for rice pudding or warm millet cereal that is fast and easy.

For lunch, we do mostly leftovers, salad, or canned salmon (instead of tuna) on sandwiches or more often on corn tortilla chips or lettuce.

And it truly only takes a few minutes on Saturday or Sunday to take a look at your list of foods you love, plug in some meals and pull together a shopping list. Done and done.

## The Secret of Bringing Your Own Food

A big part of setting yourself up for success is in the secret of bringing your own food with you whenever possible. There are a great number of reasons to do this, particularly when you are just starting your gluten-free journey.

---

### Time Saving Tip!

I highly recommend an app like Wunderlist for keeping your shopping list on your phone. It is easy to use and you can share one list with the whole family. So whoever can make it to the store is sure to have the full up-to-date list of what is needed for the week!

---

Primarily, it ensures that you will have something gluten free to eat, but it also means you get to be in charge of what you eat instead of being reduced to choosing between a salad and a salad.

Don't get me wrong, I love salad, but when it's the only option you have, it doesn't feel like much of a choice. Bringing your own food also reduces your risk of cheating because the decision has already been made.

Now, what exactly do I mean by "bring your own food"? Does this mean I expect you to turn your world upside-down and spend all your time in the kitchen? Will you never get to eat out?

No, I don't expect you to totally change how you live and you shouldn't expect that of yourself either. What you should be striving for is to make sure you are planning ahead. Setting yourself up for success in this instance can be easy. It may be as simple as carrying a gluten-free bar in your purse, car or briefcase.

Lunch at the office can be leftovers packed up the night before or a big salad topped with beans, canned salmon or leftover meat, rice or quinoa. Or make a dish on Sunday and eat it throughout the week. Lunch on the run might mean that you pack your lunch in a little cooler or insulated bag.

Going to a friend's house for dinner is best approached by letting the host know you would like to bring a dish to share. Bringing your own food doesn't have to be hard or keep you tied to the kitchen--it just needs to be something that you give some thought to because it really will make a difference in how you feel and how you succeed.

## Tips on Eating Out

Eating out can be a challenge. Not only is it one of the more common times that people cheat, but also you will have to look out for the many hidden sources of gluten in restaurant foods.

For instance, french fries seem safe, but they almost always have flour on them and even when they don't they're cooked in the same oil as all of the other breaded, deep-fried treats--I mean menu items. All that said, if you go out armed with a great mindset and these guidelines you will succeed!

If you are on a strict no gluten diet you really should stick to restaurants that have a dedicated gluten-free kitchen. There is a great resource for this available at:
www.findmeglutenfree.com

On this site, and their available app, you can search for restaurants in your area with gluten-free menu items or you can filter for dedicated gluten-free facilities.

If you aren't as concerned about cross-contamination, here is a website where you can find a list of gluten-free dishes from around the world. It is helpful for determining what foods you

can eat when dining out:
www.gluten-free-around-the-world.com

And, here are some simple tips to give you a good starting point.

Some generally safe options:

- Salads without croutons or breaded meats (you may need to watch out for the dressing, I usually opt for a vinaigrette)
- Non-breaded whole food dishes such as grilled chicken breast, fish or steak with steamed veggies or rice are really your best bet. (You will need to look out for marinades, gravies and soy sauce)
- Mexican food (You will want to avoid the flour tortillas and fried items)

Best to avoid:

- Gravy and other sauces
- Sausages
- Meatloaf
- Burgers (unless you are sure they are made from real ground beef)
- Soups
- Casseroles
- Chinese food

These are the guidelines that I live by, but you will need to do your own research and ask lots of questions so that you know more about restaurants and ingredients near you. And, of course, be sure to use your best judgement when deciding when and where to eat out.

# CHAPTER 6

## DEALING WITH NAYSAYERS

AKA Family and Friends

Gluten and following a gluten-free diet can be controversial conversation topics. This may not be something you have ever experienced. Maybe you have found a way to surround yourself with open-minded understanding people who support your every decision. If that is the case, stop reading for a moment of silence and be thankful.

For most, though you may have wonderful supportive friends, you will likely run into or be related to someone who will ridicule you, even if only as a joke. And even the most well-intentioned friends and family may not fully understand why you are going gluten free. Whether they are snarky, mean or just don't understand, it will happen and here's how to handle it.

In my experience there are four types of people you will encounter: The Know It All, The Snarky Ones, The Clueless and The Well Intentioned.

## The Know It All

You've met these folks. They're the type of people who have an opinion on everything and aren't afraid to share it. They boldly speak their mind though rarely have they done any real research to formulate that opinion. There are two ways to deal with those who think they know it all:

1. Do not engage. Let them spout off their unfounded beliefs and know that they aren't really interested in your point of view, your experience or the truth. If they were, they would have asked. In this case, sometimes it is just easier to know your truth, save your breath and go on about your merry way.

2. Let 'em have it. If you are dealing with someone who you think might be open to hearing your point of view--maybe someone close to you--or if you enjoy a good debate, by all means, share what you know and make it good.

## The Snarky Ones

The folks who like to joke or make unnecessary comments about your food choices are usually the type of people who are either in the habit of putting people down to feel good about themselves or they just like to hear their own voices. Either way not much thought seems to go into what comes out of their mouths.

With these folks I tend to just let it go. I personally don't find it worthwhile to engage them. I just can't find the good in it. If, however, what they say is particularly hurtful or if it is someone that you see often, have a quick heart-to-heart. Explain that this is something you feel you must do to improve your health and that you don't appreciate his or her comments. I've found that with most people when you open up, they shut up.

## The Clueless

People who ask silly questions or seem completely clueless simply have no idea. They truly aren't making fun of you. They are often just trying to understand a bit about you or make small talk. Don't fret about it or over-analyze it. Simply answer their question and move on about your day.

## The Well Intentioned

These are the caring people in your life who try to do their best to take your dietary needs into account, but don't always hit the mark. They want you to feel included, but they really don't know the first thing about gluten.

They may bake cookies with half gluten-free flour and half wheat flour. Or they'll make a rice dish because *rice is safe, right?* But then cover it in soy sauce because, *how much gluten could be in that?* They might even invite you over, and after insisting that you should not bring your own food, you arrive to find that there is not a single solitary thing that you can eat.

What do you do? First, you stop and take the time to be thankful. This person obviously loves you and just wants to spend time with you and make you feel included. And be sure that you don't keep those thanks to yourself. Tell them how much you appreciate their efforts. Then when things are calm and you have some time to talk, explain what you can in a way they'll understand. Give them enough information without burying them in the details. Be sure to ask if they have any questions and answer them the best way you can.

Finally, offer to help. Insist on bringing your own food or a potluck dish to share. It may help to say that you are still experimenting with gluten-free recipes yourself and can use the practice. Besides, what really matters is that you get to spend time together.

Now that you have some ammo on how to deal with those who may question your choices, let's talk about food!! In the next chapter you will find the recipes that I believe are absolutely essential to making your journey to a gluten-free life a huge success!

# CHAPTER 7

## ABSOLUTELY ESSENTIAL GLUTEN-FREE BAKING RECIPES

T his selection of recipes will make your transition to gluten free exponentially easier. From bread and pizza dough to muffins, pancakes and cookies--you are guaranteed to have great food to help you through. To get started we must first learn a bit about gluten-free flours.

## A Discussion on Gluten-Free Flours

The challenge with gluten-free flour is, quite obviously, the lack of gluten. Gluten is what gives wheat flour its structure as well as its ability to rise and hold air. It's the gluten that gives baked goods their soft yet chewy consistency. So, the biggest challenge in gluten-free baking is to find a suitable substitute for wheat flour and the gluten it contains.

There are a myriad of ways to blend different flours, starches and gums together in hopes of the perfect balance. Which is why gluten-free all-purpose flours are not created equal. Although most will do a fine job and result in edible baked goods, if you really want to be successful you want to have food that is more than just edible. You want it to be delicious!

For this reason, the flour that you choose really does matter. Some people go so far as to create different flour blends for different baked goods. That is great if you have the time, but I am here to help you get started and to help make your transition to a gluten-free life easier. So, I am going to focus on how to choose a good gluten-free flour blend that will work quite well for all of your basic baking needs.

When choosing a gluten-free all-purpose flour you want to look for one that has the following characteristics:

- At least some brown rice flour or other whole grain flour (it will say "whole grain ____" on the list of ingredients)
- White rice flour should be near the top of the list of ingredients
- Starches such as potato, tapioca or corn starch should be further down the ingredients list
- Xanthan gum, guar gum or acacia gum can either be present or not. (Keep in mind that if one of these gums is present in your flour you will omit xanthan gum from any recipe that calls for it.)

---

### What Is Xanthan Gum Exactly?

It is a common food additive that makes things like salad dressing and ice cream blend more smoothly. It is made when corn sugar is fermented by the same bacteria that makes the black spots on cauliflower. And in gluten-free baking, we use it as a replacement for the gluten. It helps make the dough sticky.

---

If your gluten-free flour blend includes xanthan, guar or acacia gum you can omit the xanthan gum from any recipe that calls for it.

So, which gluten-free flour blends do I recommend?

- Pamela's (my favorite)
- Bob's Red Mill Gluten-Free 1:1 Baking Flour
- Better Batter All-Purpose Flour Mix
- King Arthur Gluten-Free Measure for Measure Flour

Pamela's brand gluten-free flour blend is my favorite because not only is it a great flour that bakes up well and tastes great, but it also doesn't contain any of the ingredients that are commonly a problem for people with multiple food allergies. Of course, if you do have multiple food allergies, consult the label to be sure it is safe for you.

If you are interested in more information on gluten-free flour, what purpose all of the components serve and how to build your own gluten-free flour blend, I highly suggest both of these books. They are full of great information and lots of wonderful recipes:

- Gluten Free On A Shoestring Bakes Bread by Nicole Hunn
- The How Can It Be Gluten Free Cookbook by America's Test Kitchen

## Measuring Your Flour Correctly

Surely, you think I'm joking. Of course you know how to measure flour. I know it sounds nuts, but I am not joking. Hear me out and you'll see why I bring it up.

I really disliked baking for years. It was time consuming, messy and my baked goods were inconsistent at best. At worst, they turned out dense, dry and flavorless except for that hint of burnt--and that was with wheat flour!

Occasionally, I was able to bake something that was really amazing, like the lemon chiffon cake I made from scratch for my grandma's birthday. But, it happened so infrequently that I really wasn't interested in baking, ever. In my mind, baking was an act of futility and my time could be better spent doing--basically anything else. Besides, the available commercial products were tasty and affordable.

When we went gluten free however, all that changed. Not only were the gluten-free versions of our staples not affordable, but they tasted awful. If we were going to make it on this path, it became apparent that I needed to change my outlook on baking.

THE ESSENTIAL GLUTEN-FREE GUIDE

So, I started searching for gluten-free recipes with excellent reviews. It seemed no matter what I searched for these three blogs kept coming up consistently:

- Gluten Free On A Shoestring
- The Minimalist Baker
- My Whole Food Life

These blogs changed my outlook on baking and ultimately made my gluten-free journey a success.

I also turned for help to my favorite cooking resource-- America's Test Kitchen (ATK). ATK is known for breaking down recipes and creating the ultimate version of that recipe. I have literally never had a recipe of theirs that did not turn out or that my whole family didn't love.

When I was searching for ways to improve my baking, it was well before ATK had even dabbled in the gluten-free arena. But I had had such great success with them in the past, so I went looking in their regular baking books for tips. I was floored. There it was. The key to my baking disasters. It was in how I was measuring my flour!

You see, flour compacts and when you use the measuring cup to scoop up the flour you get tons of variation in how much flour is being scooped leading to inconsistent results and often dry, dense baked goods.

All this is to say, when you measure flour use a spoon to scoop the flour, sprinkle it into your dry measuring cup until heaping and then use the back of a butter knife to scrape off the excess flour. This is the first and probably the most important step in making baked goods that you will be proud to share.

Now that we have the flour and technique covered, let's get to the recipes! The recipes in this chapter are the ones that I consider absolutely essential to transitioning to a gluten-free diet. Let's dig in.

For printable versions of these and all included recipes visit: www.healthyana.net/essentialgf

## The Best Gluten-Free Bread Recipes

Bread that tastes like real bread is an absolute must for making the gluten-free transition. There is only one way to get it that I have found--you have to make it.

STOP right there and take a good, long deep breath. I promise it's going to be okay. You are going to at least consider doing this because, remember, you have a great, really deep "why" behind your decision to go gluten free. And guess what, it's really a breeze. You can do this!!

The easiest way is to use a bread mix for your bread. These two are awesome!

- Pamela's Gluten-Free Bread Mix.
- King Arthur Gluten-Free Bread Mix

I have yet to find another gluten-free flour blend that works as well these. Both are available on Amazon and in most "natural" grocery stores. Pamela's® Bread Mix happens to be my favorite mostly because I have more experience with it.

Pamela's is a much better value than the King Arthur® bread mix. Pamela's® should be between $11 and $16 for a four-pound bag (as of the printing of this book). I know that sounds like a lot when compared to regular flour, but compared to the price of gluten-free bread, it's a steal. King Arthur's® bread mix is just under $10 for an 18 ounce box - which makes one loaf or 2 pizza crusts. It is definitely pricier, but if that is what you can get your hands on it does make a tasty loaf! And it tastes a million times better than so many store-bought gluten-free breads. Plus, it's easy and makes a beautiful and delicious loaf that even your gluten-loving inner gremlin will approve of.

## The Best Gluten-Free Sandwich Bread
Makes 1 loaf

## INGREDIENTS:
- 3½ cups gluten-free flour blend - specifically for breads
- 2¼ tsp. active dry yeast or 1 yeast packet 7g
- 2 large eggs

- 1/3 cup oil
- 1¼ cups + 1 Tbs. warm water

## BREAD MACHINE DIRECTIONS:
- Pour water and oil into bread machine.
- Add eggs.
- Add flour on top of liquid.
- Create a crater in the center of the flour and add the yeast there. Take care that the yeast does not touch the liquid below the flour.
- Start bread machine using the following settings: Basic White Bread and Medium Crust. (If your machine has a gluten-free setting DO NOT use it. It doesn't turn out.)
- Be sure to scrape down the sides of the bread pan part way through mixing.
- When the bread is done, remove from pan immediately.
- Place on a wire rack and allow to cool completely before slicing.

## OVEN BAKING DIRECTIONS:
- Lightly grease a loaf pan and set aside.
- Place flour and yeast in a large mixing bowl.
- In a small bowl, mix 1/3 cup oil, eggs, and warm water until combined.
- Add the wet ingredients to the mixing bowl and mix on high for 3 minutes.

THE ESSENTIAL GLUTEN-FREE GUIDE

- Transfer dough to prepared loaf pan and let dough rest for 60 to 90 minutes.
- Take care that the dough is not in a draft.
- Dough may not rise much during this time, and that's okay.
- Preheat oven to 350°F.
- Bake for 60 to 70 minutes until golden brown and firm to the touch.
- Allow to cool for 10 minutes in the loaf pan.
- Transfer from pan to wire rack.
- Allow to cool completely before slicing.

Slice bread only as you use it and store in plastic in the refrigerator.

## The Best Gluten-Free Soda Bread
(Also yeast-free, dairy-free and egg-free)
Makes 1 loaf

### INGREDIENTS:
3½ cups gluten-free flour blend (a bread blend works best)
1¼ tsp. xanthan gum (omit if your flour blend includes it)
½ tsp. sea salt
1 tsp. baking soda
1¾ cups coconut or cashew milk (whole milk works too)
1 Tbs. + 3 tsp. apple cider vinegar
1 Tbs. honey
Optional: 1 Tbs. fresh chopped herbs (rosemary or thyme)

## DIRECTIONS:

- Preheat oven to 425°F.
- Measure out nut milk and add the apple cider vinegar. Stir and allow to sit at least 5 mins.
- Mix all dry ingredients in one bowl.
- Mix wet ingredients into milk mixture.
- Then add wet ingredients to dry and mix until combined.
- The batter may seem like it is too wet. If you find it too hard to work with put it into the freezer for 10 minutes so it better holds its shape.
- Dust the batter with just a little extra GF flour and quickly form batter into ball and place on parchment paper covered cookie sheet or baking stone.
- Cut an X in the top of the loaf about ¼" deep with serrated bread knife.
- Bake for 20 minutes then rotate pan.
- Continue to bake for 20-25 mins. until loaf is golden brown and firm to the touch.
- Allow to cool completely before slicing. Only slice as you eat it and store in plastic.

## The Best Gluten-Free Orange-Cranberry Soda Bread

(Also yeast-free, dairy-free and egg-free)
Makes 1 loaf

## INGREDIENTS:

3½ cups gluten-free all-purpose flour (bread blend is best)

1¼ tsp. xanthan gum (omit if your blend includes it)

½ tsp. sea salt

1 tsp. baking soda

Zest of 1 orange

1¾ cups coconut or cashew milk (whole milk works too)

1 Tbs. + 3 tsp. apple cider vinegar

2 Tbs. honey

1 cup dried cranberries

## DIRECTIONS:

- Preheat oven to 425°F.
- Measure out nut milk and add the apple cider vinegar. Stir and allow to sit at least 5 mins.
- Mix all dry ingredients in one bowl.
- Mix wet ingredients into milk mixture.
- Then add wet ingredients to dry and mix until combined.
- Fold in dried cranberries.
- The batter may seem like it is too wet. If you find it too hard to work with put it into the freezer for 10 minutes so it better holds its shape.
- Dust the batter with just a little extra GF flour and quickly form batter into ball and place on parchment paper covered cookie sheet or baking stone.
- Cut an X in the top of the loaf about ¼" deep with serrated bread knife.

- Bake for 20 minutes then rotate pan.
- Continue to bake for 20-25 mins. until loaf is golden brown and firm to the touch.
- Allow to cool completely before slicing.
- Slice as you eat it and store in plastic.

# Easy Gluten-Free Pizza Crust Recipe

Next to bread, the thing I hear most often that people miss when going gluten free is good pizza. This dough is absolutely the best version I have found, including any store-bought or restaurant pizzas I have tried. And again--no gluten, no kneading! Spread it out and let it rise--it's that easy!

## The Best Gluten-Free Pizza Dough
Makes (2) 12" pizza crusts

### INGREDIENTS:
3½ cups gluten-free flour blend - specifically for breads
2¼ tsp. active dry yeast or 1 yeast packet 7g
¼ cup olive oil
1½ cups warm water
2 tsp. oregano (optional)

### DIRECTIONS:
- Cover 2 cookie sheets with parchment paper.
- Combine all ingredients in a large mixing bowl.
- Mix on medium for 2 minutes until dough is smooth.
- Transfer ½ of the dough to one of the parchment

paper lined cookie sheets.
- Use the oiled palm of your hand to gently smooth dough into pizza crust shape. Add additional oil, preferably olive oil, as needed to prevent sticking.
- Shape the dough into as large or small, thick or thin as you would like. The dough will rise to about twice as thick.
- Close up any holes made as you go.
- Repeat the shaping process for the second crust.
- Allow dough to sit and rise for 1 hour.
- Place rack in top third of oven and preheat oven to 375°F.
- When oven comes to temperature place dough in the oven.
- Bake crust for 8 to 10 minutes, until hint of brown. (A little longer for thicker crusts.)
- If you are cooking both crusts at the same time rotate them ½ way through baking time. And it may take a little longer for the crusts to begin to brown.
- While crust is baking, pre-cook any meats or vegetables that require cooking as topping will only be warmed through in final bake.

MAKE AHEAD OPTION: wrap and freeze par-baked crusts for later use.

## Add the toppings:
- Preheat oven to 450°F.
- Add sauce and toppings to the crust.
- Once oven comes to temperature bake for an additional 5 to 10 minutes until cheese is bubbly and just beginning to brown.

## Gluten-Free Pancake & Waffle Recipes

Everyone needs a go-to pancake and/or waffle recipe for those lazy Sunday mornings. Certainly, you could buy Pamela's, Arrowhead Mills or King Arthur brand gluten-free pancake mix, but for anyone who likes to keep their pantry simple, as I do, here are two reliable recipes:

## "Go-to" Gluten-Free Pancakes
Makes (12-16) pancakes

### INGREDIENTS:
2 cups gluten-free all-purpose flour blend
3 tsp. baking powder
2¼ cups coconut or cashew milk (whole milk works too)
2 eggs
3 Tbs. butter (melted and cooled) or oil (mild flavored is best)
1 tsp. vanilla extract

### DIRECTIONS:
- Mix all dry ingredients in one bowl.
- Mix wet ingredients in a separate bowl until combined.

THE ESSENTIAL GLUTEN-FREE GUIDE

- Then add wet ingredients to dry and mix until combined.
- Preheat skillet with 1 teaspoon oil or butter.
- Add additional water or nut milk ¼ cup at a time to thin batter if it is a little too thick.  Mix thoroughly between each addition.
- Pour ~¼ cup of batter onto hot skillet.
- Allow to cook without turning until bubbles at the edges pop and the cake edge is firm.
- Flip and cook until golden brown and cooked through.

Enjoy warm with syrup or your choice of toppings!


## Wondrous Gluten-Free Waffles
Makes 8 standard waffles

### INGREDIENTS:
1¼ cups gluten-free all-purpose flour blend
½ tsp. baking powder
1 tsp. baking soda
1¼ cup coconut or cashew milk (whole milk works too)
2 tsp. white vinegar
2 eggs
2 Tbs. butter (melted and cooled) or oil (mild flavored)

## DIRECTIONS:

- Measure out nut milk and add the vinegar. Stir and allow to sit at least 5 mins.
- Mix all dry ingredients in one bowl.
- Mix wet ingredients into milk mixture.
- Then add wet ingredients to dry and mix with whisk until combined.
- Add water or nut milk to thin batter if it is a little too thick.
- Preheat waffle iron and grease with oil or butter.
- Pour batter onto hot waffle iron.
- Allow to cook until light golden brown.

Note: They take longer than traditional waffles to cook. And the batter may thicken as it sits. You can add water or nut milk to thin the batter if it gets too thick.

Enjoy warm with syrup or your choice of toppings!

## Gluten-Free Muffin & Scone Recipes

Muffins and scones have become a pretty big part of our life since going gluten free. They work for breakfast, snacks or even dessert. Here are a couple of our favorites:

## Gluten-Free Banana Chocolate Chip Muffins
Makes 12 muffins

### INGREDIENTS:
1¾ cups gluten-free all-purpose flour blend
¼ tsp. xanthan gum (omit if your blend already contains it)
1 Tbs. baking powder
½ tsp. cinnamon
¼ tsp. sea salt
3 bananas (the more ripe and spotted the better)
¼ cup cashew or coconut milk (whole milk works too)
2 eggs
¼ cup maple syrup
3 Tbs. honey
1 tsp. vanilla extract
½ cup mini chocolate chips

### DIRECTIONS:
- Preheat oven to 350°F.
- Mix dry ingredients in one bowl.
- Mix wet in another bowl.
- Add dry to wet and mix until combined.
- Fold in the chocolate chips.
- Spoon mixture into lined muffin pans.
- Bake for 18-22 minutes.
- Let the muffins cool completely before removing them from the pans.

Store in the fridge. You can also freeze them for longer storage! Enjoy!

# Gluten-Free Blueberry Muffins

Makes 12 muffins

*good!*

*didn't use*

## INGREDIENTS:

2 cups gluten-free all-purpose flour blend

¼ tsp. xanthan gum (omit if your blend already includes it)

2 tsp. baking powder

½ tsp. sea salt

Zest of ½ lemon

1 tsp. vanilla extract

½ cup maple syrup

½ cup coconut or cashew milk (whole milk works too)

4 ~~5~~ Tbs. butter, melted and cooled

2 eggs

1 heaping cup blueberries (fresh or frozen)

## DIRECTIONS:

- Preheat oven to 350°F.
- Mix all dry ingredients in one bowl.
- Take a tablespoon of flour mixture and add to blueberries in a separate bowl, mix to coat blueberries and set aside.
- Mix wet ingredients in another bowl.
- Then add wet ingredients to dry and mix until combined.
- Fold in the blueberries.
- Spoon batter into lined muffin pans.
- Bake for about 18-22 minutes or until a toothpick

comes out clean.
- Wait until muffins are completely cooled before removing from pans.

Store in the fridge or freezer. Enjoy!

## Gluten-Free Pumpkin Cranberry Muffins
Makes 24 muffins

### INGREDIENTS:
2 cups gluten-free all-purpose flour blend
½ tsp. xanthan gum (omit if your blend includes it)
1 tsp. baking powder
1 tsp. baking soda
½ tsp. sea salt
1 Tbs. + 2 tsp. cinnamon
1 tsp. cloves
1 can pumpkin puree
¼ cup coconut milk (whole milk works too)
4 eggs
½ cup honey
¼ cup coconut sugar (packed)
½ cup butter, melted and cooled
1 tsp. vanilla
1½ cup dried cranberries
zest from 1 orange

## DIRECTIONS:

- Preheat oven to 350°F.
- Mix dry ingredients in one bowl.
- Mix wet in another bowl.
- Add dry to wet and mix until combined.
- Fold in the dried cranberries.
- Spoon mixture into lined muffin pans.
- Bake for 18-25 minutes or until toothpick comes out clean.
- Let the muffins cool completely before removing them from the pans.

Store in the fridge or freezer.  Enjoy!

## Gluten-Free Cinnamon Apple Scones
(dairy-free and egg-free)
Makes 8 scones

## INGREDIENTS:
2 Gala or Fuji apples, peeled, cored and diced
1 Tbs. cinnamon
1 Tbs. sugar
2 cups gluten-free all-purpose flour blend
½ tsp. xanthan gum (omit if your blend includes it)
1 Tbs. of baking powder
½ tsp. sea salt
3 Tbs. sugar
5 Tbs. butter, diced and chilled
1 cup cashew or coconut milk, chilled (whole milk works too)

## DIRECTIONS:

- Preheat oven to 400°F.
- Mix diced apples in cinnamon and 1 Tbs. of sugar, set aside.
- Mix dry ingredients in food processor until combined.
- Add butter and pulse 10 times for 1 second each.
- Move the mixture to a large mixing bowl.
- Quickly add the chilled milk and stir just until dough starts to come together.
- Fold in the prepared apples.
- Turn out onto parchment covered plate and flatten to less than 2" thick.
- Place plate with dough in the freezer for 10 minutes.
- Turn chilled dough onto a parchment covered countertop.
- Quickly shape the dough into a circle about 1" thick.
- Using a knife or board scraper cut the dough into 8 equal pie pieces.
- Space the scones out with at least 1 ½" between them.
- Transfer the parchment paper to a cookie sheet.
- Bake for 18-22 mins until slightly golden brown.
- Allow to cool 10 mins and enjoy!

Store in the fridge or freezer.

## VARIATIONS:

1. Leave out the cinnamon apples and replace with ¾ cup mini chocolate chips.
2. Leave out the cinnamon apples and replace with ¾ cup sliced strawberries or blueberries (frozen works well).
3. Leave out the cinnamon apples and replace with ½ cup pitted cherries and ½ cup mini chocolate chips.

## Gluten-Free Oatmeal Scones

Makes 8 scones

## INGREDIENTS:

2 cups gluten-free all-purpose flour
1 Tbs. baking powder
¼ tsp. sea salt
6 Tbs. butter, cubed and chilled
1½ cups gluten-free rolled oats
¾ cup cashew or coconut milk (whole milk works too)
¼ cup maple syrup
1 egg

## DIRECTIONS:

- Preheat oven to 400°F.
- Whisk together milk, syrup and egg in measuring cup and set aside.
- Mix dry ingredients in food processor until combined.
- Add butter and pulse 10 times for 1 second each.

- Transfer the mixture to a large mixing bowl.
- Add the oats and mix to combine.
- Add milk mixture and fold in until dough begins to form. (dough will be thick, but wet)
- Turn out onto parchment covered plate and flatten to less than 2" thick.
- Place plate with dough in the freezer for 10 minutes.
- Turn chilled dough onto a parchment covered countertop.
- Quickly shape the dough into a circle about 1" thick.
- Using a knife or board scraper cut the dough into 8 equal pie pieces.
- Space the scones on the parchment paper with at least 1 ½" between them.
- Transfer the parchment paper to a cookie sheet.
- Bake for 18-22 mins until slightly golden brown.

## Gluten-Free Pie Crust Recipe

A gluten-free pie crust recipe is a great way to expand your meal plan options with quiche, pot pies and of course dessert! This one is not only easy to make (especially if you have a food processor), but is buttery and delicious. Plus, since this recipe is for 2 crusts it's easy to make and freeze them ahead to have on hand later!

## Gluten-Free Pie Crust Recipe
Makes 2 Crusts

### INGREDIENTS:
3 cups gluten-free all-purpose flour (bread blends work best)
1 cup butter (diced and chilled)
~8 Tbs. ice water

### DIRECTIONS:
- Cut cold butter into flour with 2 knives until smaller than pea sized pieces remain (or in food processor until mixture resembles coarse sand).
- Add chilled water 1 Tbs. at a time (mix after each addition) until dough comes together.
- Cover dough and chill for 10 minutes.
- Take ½ the dough and roll it out between two sheets of parchment paper until about ⅛" thick.
- Peel off top layer of parchment and turn over onto a lightly greased pie pan.
- Remove the second piece of parchment and mold the pie edge.
- Bake according to pie recipe.

**Note:** Dough can be made ahead and frozen for later use.

## Gluten-Free Cake Recipes and Baking from a Box

Well, I am all for it. Cakes are something that I have never had the wherewithal to make from scratch. I know some people love it and find that it is worth the work, but to me baking from a box is easier and tastes just fine.

When it comes to cake mix in a box or a bag, as the case may be, my favorite brands are:

- King Arthur
- Arrowhead Mills
- Wholesome Chow (no eggs or dairy)

Each of these brands delivers a great fluffy cake that is super easy to make and tastes great!

If you like baking cakes from scratch I would steer you to the gluten-free sites highlighted in the next chapter for recipes and I would stick to recipes that are specifically gluten free to save yourself some headaches.

And as for brownies my ultimate boxed recommendation is:

- Arrowhead Mills Gluten-Free Fudge Brownie Mix

Truly, it's amazing!

# CHAPTER 8

## CONVERTING RECIPES TO GLUTEN FREE

When making a change to your diet it is always comforting to be able to return to at least a couple of familiar recipes. Luckily, when it comes to going gluten free this is often easily accomplished with some simple substitutions.

For instance, gluten-free pasta alone saves tons of recipes. Then there's gluten-free pie crust and pizza dough, which are also lifesavers in my book. After that we will take a look at some common minor ingredients like breadcrumbs, tortillas, and soy sauce that have gluten-free counterparts which make converting recipes simple.

We will also discuss which gluten-free flour to use for sauces and gravy and why it makes such a big difference. Finally, we will dig into gluten-free baking and which substitutions work and which don't. Let's get started!

## Finding the Best Gluten-Free Bread

I know we already talked about this, but it bears repeating: great gluten-free bread will ease you into your new gluten-free lifestyle. Homemade tastes best, but in case you run out, you might want a backup loaf in your freezer. Here is a guide with our reviews of some of the more popular gluten-free bread brands out there:

- Canyon Bakehouse®--This brand is our favorite. They have sandwich bread, cinnamon raisin bread, bagels, hamburger buns and they are all top notch. If you can find this brand it is definitely my top recommendation.
- Three Bakers® - Is another good option if you can find them in your area. They also offer pre-made pizza crust and the elusive good gluten-free hot dog bun.
- Rudi's Organic Bakery® - one of the better sandwich breads. Be aware they also sell wheat bread side by side with the gluten-free options so read the label carefully.
- Dr. Schar Artisan Baker® - They do a bunch of varieties including hot dog buns and ciabatta style rolls, but their best offering by far is their baguettes which you finish baking in the oven for five minutes-- amazing!! All of the varieties are better if you warm them up a bit. Solid choice.
- Udi's Gluten Free® - I can only suggest this brand as a last resort. It is better than nothing, but leaves a lot to be desired. As with other brands, warming it up does help improve it. I must note that I know people who love Udi's; maybe I'm spoiled, but you deserve better.

## The Best Gluten-Free Pasta

Gluten-free pasta is just about the easiest substitution there is when it comes to taking recipes you already know how to make and making them gluten free. There are also many kinds of gluten-free pasta out there. Which is best?

The good news is you have lots of options and now they are available even in many conventional grocery stores--yippie! I can recommend any of the many that have corn and quinoa as main ingredients. They taste good and the consistency is very close to your average dried wheat pasta. Even my gluten loving in-laws can't tell the difference.

I would urge you to choose an organic brand which tells you that it was not made with GMO corn.

If you cannot tolerate corn, the next best thing is DeBoles® brand Gluten-Free Multigrain Spaghetti Style Pasta. It is made mostly with rice flour, but also includes amaranth and quinoa which make for better texture and it tastes great too.

I certainly have not tried all of the available gluten-free pastas, but I have found that these cook up well and have a texture that is most similar to wheat flour pasta.

In contrast, brown rice pasta has an odd consistency and is easily overcooked going from hard to chewy/mushy in what seems like an instant. I would only recommend it as a last resort.

Whichever pasta you choose, do yourself a favor and use a timer. Bring the water to a boil, add the pasta and as soon as it begins to boil again set the timer for whatever time the directions say on the box. I find that eight minutes is almost always perfect. Then drain the pasta and rinse it with cold water. This rinses the extra starch out and keeps it from continuing to cook. It really makes a difference in the final product.

## Pre-made Gluten-Free Pizza Crust

For most of us, pizza is a must, at least occasionally, so let's talk about crust. Now, I realize that most people don't make their own pizza and if frozen pizza works for you, you're in luck! There are quite a few options available.

And gluten-free pizza options at restaurants are becoming more popular. Even Domino's now has it on their menu, but because of possible cross-contamination in restaurants, the crazy prices, and the fact that these crusts are nothing to write home about, you may want to make it yourself. I know, I know, here I go again, trying to make you bake, but truly it is easy--much easier than wheat pizza dough--and so worth it! This crust is thicker, chewier and more delicious than any other gluten-free pizza dough I've had. The recipe can be found in Chapter 7.

There are also a few pre-made gluten-free crusts on the market, but they almost all contain eggs and many include dairy as well, so if you have additional food intolerances, beware. Udi's is the only one I have tried and it's pretty good if you like thin crust pizza. It can be found in the freezer section with the other frozen gluten-free breads.

## Pre-made Gluten-Free Pie Crust

Gluten-free pie crusts are great, not only for dessert pies, but for quiches and pot pies. And it is another simple substitution to keep using those recipes you love. It's easy to make yourself, if you have a food processor--otherwise it is kind of a pain. Our favorite recipe can be found in Chapter 7.

Pre-made gluten-free crusts are also available and some are quite good, from a taste and texture standpoint. (Finally! Something I can recommend that is pre-made!) My favorite is by Pillsbury. There are certainly ingredients that aren't my favorite such as non-organic cornstarch and non-organic and hydrogenated soybean oil, but if convenience is your main goal, it is easy and tasty. It comes in a tub. You just press it into a pie plate and bake your pie as directed--easy as pie!

## Easy Substitutions - Breadcrumbs, Tortillas, & Soy Sauce

Some substitutions are very simple--for instance, gluten-free breadcrumbs are available commercially. The brand that I use is Aleia's and it works well to substitute in everything from breaded chicken or fish to meatloaf and casseroles. Use it as an exact substitute and it should work well. If you cannot find gluten-free breadcrumbs at your local store, they can be found online through Amazon.com as of the printing of this book.

And of course if you'd like you can save some money and make them yourself by toasting gluten-free bread in a 300 degree oven for 10-15 minutes, turning halfway through. Then run through a food processor until the desired consistency is reached.

Gluten-free Mexican food at home is a cinch as there are not many cereal grains to replace. Often the only substitutions you need to make is to switch from flour tortillas to corn or you can use gluten-free flour tortillas that are now available commercially, super easy and they taste great!

Asian cuisine is difficult if not impossible to get gluten free when eating out, but it can be made at home. You will have to switch to a gluten-free soy sauce such as Tamari® or you could use Bragg's Liquid Amino Acids® in place of soy sauce. It tastes a little different, but is gluten free, non-GMO and has amino acids that are important to replace especially in a vegetarian or vegan diet. Coconut Aminos is another alternative to soy sauce that is gluten free and soy free and tastes a little sweet, less salty.

Depending on what you are making you may also need gluten-free oyster sauce, Wok Mei® offers one and Kikkoman®

makes a gluten-free hoisin sauce. Both are available online and at most "natural" grocery stores.

And though most should be safe you will have to look at the labels on noodles, wrappers and other sauces.

## The Secret to Gluten-Free Sauces, Gravy & Fried Chicken

This is one area where gluten-free flour beats regular wheat flour (yay!) when used as a thickener or for dredging. Here's why: if you have ever made sauce or gravy before and had to whisk that hot liquid like crazy to keep lumps from forming in the sauce you know that it can be a real arm killer.

As it turns out, gluten is what causes lumps in your gravy. It is also what can make your fried chicken a little gummy if the oil wasn't quite hot enough. Gluten is obviously an integral part of wheat flour so when you cook with it, you are just kind of stuck with it. But when you are gluten free, you have options.

We are generally trying to add items into gluten-free flour to make it mimic gluten and generally those things are xanthan gum or guar gum. So, in this case you can just leave them out or use a gluten-free flour blend that does not have the xanthan gum in it for a lump-free gravy. Bob's Red Mill® has one and I'm sure there are others out there. Or if you would prefer potato flour also works great as a thickener. So, finally we found something that gluten free can do better!

# 1:1 Substitutions in Gluten-Free Baking

The question is, can you take your grandma's famous banana bread recipe and substitute only the flour for a gluten-free blend without changing the rest of the recipe? The answer, is decidedly--almost never.

The bottom line is 1:1 substitutions can work, but they rarely work perfectly. It really depends on how much effort you want to put into tweaking the recipe, which usually involves reducing the fat (butter/oil) by about one-third, and increasing the eggs (usually by 1) or adding additional liquid in the form of milk.

You may find that when baking gluten free, it helps to use a vetted gluten-free recipe to maximize your success. Some of my favorite places to find fool-proof gluten-free recipes are:

America's Test Kitchen - Though their content online requires a membership they have a few great gluten-free cookbooks with all the tips you need to help you convert recipes you love and hundreds of recipes that work and taste great every time. www.americastestkitchen.com

Gluten Free On a Shoestring - Nicole started her blog seven years ago to share gluten-free recipes with others and now has four cookbooks available! Her recipes are easy and delicious. www.glutenfreeonashoestring.com

Minimalist Baker - Most of the recipes here are gluten free, but not all of them so take care. Dana highlights recipes that are simple with few ingredients and that only require one bowl. She also does not use dairy or eggs in her cooking so people with multiple food allergies will love her. Her recipes are awesome and she has two cookbooks!
www.minimalistbaker.com

My Whole Food Life - Not all of the recipes on this site are gluten free, but many are and it is a great resource for quick and easy recipes for real food.
www.mywholefoodlife.com

Elana's Pantry - The recipes on this blog are paleo, completely grain-free, and super delicious. Elana gave up grains in 2001 and now has three cookbooks!
www.elanaspantry.com

No Gluten, No Problem - Pete and Kelli Bronski, are a husband-and-wife team that cook up some amazing gluten-free recipes. They too have four cookbooks with rave reviews!
www.nogluten-noproblem.com

There are many more sites online, but I try to stick with just a handful that I know will have recipes that really work for me.

# CHAPTER 9

## MORE GLUTEN-FREE RECIPES

Have you ever met a vegetarian who doesn't actually eat vegetables? I have met quite a few and somehow it always surprises me. They've removed the meat from their diet and generally have replaced it with meat-like alternatives--veggie burgers, veggie chicken patties and more. This happens because they took the first step of cutting out the meat, but stopped there.

When it comes to transitioning to a gluten-free diet people often do the same thing. They search for and find gluten-free alternatives to foods that generally contain gluten. This is absolutely fine and to be expected. It is part of the process. However, as you progress on your gluten-free journey you may find that you aren't as satisfied with your food options. You may find that broadening your horizons and trying new dishes that inherently don't contain gluten can be freeing. It's like opening a whole new dimension of culinary greatness.

For this reason, I have selected a mixture of recipes that cover both of these categories. Some have been adapted to be gluten free and others that are gluten free without any adaptation. I hope that this may give you a starting point in your journey to finding a new way of eating.

For printable versions of these and all included recipes visit: www.healthyana.net/essentialgf

## Breakfast Recipes

Muffins, scones, pancakes and waffles are great for breakfast, and those recipes can be found in Chapter 7. Here are some additional tasty and make-ahead options for those busy mornings.

## Refrigerator Oats - base recipe
Single serving size

### INGREDIENTS:
½ cup gluten-free rolled oats
¾ cup milk or nut milk of your choice
¼ tsp. seasoning of choice
½ cup chopped fruit (fresh or frozen)
Optional: ½ tsp. flax, chia or hemp seed
Optional: drizzle maple syrup

### DIRECTIONS:
- Add oats, milk, seasoning and any optional ingredients to airtight container.
- Mix to combine.
- Top with fruit.
- Cover and refrigerate overnight.
- Serve warm or cold with a drizzle of maple syrup.

Make a week's worth and have breakfast ready all week!

**VARIATIONS:**

1. Peaches, vanilla extract and 1 tsp. maple syrup
2. Apples, cinnamon and hemp seed
3. Blueberry, ¼ tsp. Lemon zest and 1 tsp. maple syrup
4. Cherry, almond extract and 1 Tbs. of shredded coconut
5. Strawberries, vanilla extract and 1 tsp. maple syrup

## Slow and Easy Gluten-Free Oatmeal
Serves 6

### INGREDIENTS:
5 cups water
1½ cups gluten-free steel cut oats
½ cup maple syrup
1 tsp. cinnamon
4 apples, cored and diced

### DIRECTIONS:
- Combine all ingredients in the crock pot.
- Cook on low for 6-10 hours.
- Comes out best if you stir every 45-60 mins or so.

Make it on Sunday and have it ready to heat up all week!

### VARIATIONS:
1. Top with raisins and chopped walnuts.
2. Leave out cinnamon and apples, and reduce maple syrup to 1/3 cup. Add chopped fresh or frozen strawberries and 1 tsp. of vanilla in the last hour of cooking.

Recipe courtesy of my good friend, Maura Higgins.

## Simple Gluten-Free Granola
Makes 16 servings

### INGREDIENTS:
3 cups gluten-free rolled oats
½ cup chopped almonds
½ cup pumpkin seeds
½ cup sunflower seeds
½ cup hemp seeds
½ cup gluten-free all purpose flour blend
⅛ tsp. salt
½ tsp. cinnamon
1/3 cup butter, melted and cooled
½ cup maple syrup
1 tsp. vanilla

### DIRECTIONS:
- Preheat oven to 300°F.
- Mix dry ingredients in a large bowl.
- Mix butter, syrup and vanilla in a separate bowl.
- Add wet to dry and fold together using a spatula until combined.
- Spread mixture onto an ungreased cookie sheet.
- Bake for 60 minutes turning granola with a metal spatula every 15 minutes.
- Once evenly browned remove from oven and allow to cool completely.

Store in an airtight container. And serve with yogurt or milk and top with fresh, frozen or even dried fruit.

# Wild Rice Porridge

Serves 4

## INGREDIENTS:

2 cups cooked wild rice (any leftover rice will do)

1 cup nut milk or regular milk

1 tsp. vanilla

½ tsp. cinnamon

## DIRECTIONS:

- Combine rice, milk and cinnamon in a saucepan.
- Bring to a boil over medium heat.
- Simmer 5-10 minutes until mixture is thick and milk is creamy.
- Remove from heat.
- Stir in vanilla.
- Cover and let stand 5 minutes.
- Drizzle with maple syrup, optional.

Whenever you make rice for dinner, make extra for breakfast!!

## VARIATIONS:

1. Apple Pie Rice Porridge:
   Add 1 apple peeled, cored and diced along with vanilla when you remove it from the heat.
2. Apple Banana Rice Porridge:
   Add a mashed banana and apple along with vanilla when you remove it from the heat, to thicken it up and add another dimension of flavor.

3.  Cherry Apple Rice Porridge:
    Replace cinnamon with ¼ cup fresh or frozen chopped
    and pitted cherries.

## Snacks Recipes

Some of the best snack foods are inherently gluten free: fruit with nut butter, hard boiled eggs, veggies with bean dip and trail mix to name a few. These are the best because with a mix of fiber filled-fruits and veggies and protein in nuts or beans you will feel full faster and stay satisfied longer than eating just chips or crackers. And on that note, here are some great recipes for some protein-filled make-ahead snacks.

### Snack Bars
Makes 12 bars

**INGREDIENTS:**
2 cups gluten-free rolled oats
1 cup sunflower butter (or any quality nut butter)
14 pitted dates
½ cup honey
2 Tbs. coconut oil
1 Tbs. cinnamon
½ cup pumpkin seeds
½ cup mini-chocolate chips

**DIRECTIONS:**
- Add rolled oats to food processor and pulse for 5 times for one second each.
- Add everything except the pumpkin seeds and chocolate chips.
- Pulse until well incorporated, about 45 seconds.

- Add pumpkin seeds and chocolate chips and pulse until just combined, about 5 quick pulses.
- Press dough firmly into a greased 9" x 9" pan.
- Cover and refrigerate for 15-30 minutes.
- Cut into bars.

Store in an airtight container in refrigerator for up to a week.

# Energy Balls

Makes 12 balls

## INGREDIENTS:

1 ½ cups raw cashews

1 cup unsweetened shredded coconut

½ cup dried cranberries

8 pitted dates

1 Tbs. coconut oil

1 Tbs. orange juice

## DIRECTIONS:

- Run cashews in food processor for one minute.
- Add remaining ingredients.
- Mix until a dough forms.
- Roll dough into 1-1 ½ inch balls and place in an airtight container with space between the balls.
- Use parchment paper between layers if you choose to stack them.
- Refrigerate for 15 minutes to set.

You can store them in the refrigerator for up to 2 weeks, but ours never last more than a few days!

## VARIATION:

1. Leave out dried cranberries and orange juice and replace with dried blueberries and lemon juice.

Adapted from my favorite www.mywholefoodlife.com bar recipe, Pineapple Coconut Cake Larabars.

# Almond Butter Cookie Bars

Makes 16 bars

## INGREDIENTS:

2 cup whole almonds

16 dates

½ tsp. sea salt

2 tsp. coconut oil

## DIRECTIONS:

- Line a 9" x 9" baking dish with parchment paper leaving ends long on two sides.
- Run whole almonds in food processor for 10 one second pulses.
- Add dates, salt and coconut oil in food processor until mixture starts to hold together, about 2 minutes.
- Press mixture into parchment lined baking dish.
- Allow to cool in fridge for 30 mins.
- Cut into bars.
- Using the parchment paper ends, lift the bars out of the baking dish.

Store in airtight container in the fridge.

# Roasted Cauliflower Bites

Serves 4

## INGREDIENTS:

1 cauliflower
2 Tbs. olive oil
¼ tsp. smoked Paprika
½ tsp. chile Powder
½ tsp. cumin
½ tsp. garlic Powder

## DIRECTIONS:

- Core the cauliflower and place on cutting board core side down.
- Slice the head into ¾" slices.
- Place slices and pieces that invariably fall off onto unlined, ungreased cookie sheet.
- Drizzle olive oil evenly over cauliflower.
- Add spices to a small bowl and mix to combine.
- Sprinkle spices evenly over cauliflower.
- Roast for 15 minutes then flip the cauliflower over.
- Continue roasting for an additional 15-20 minutes until edges begin brown and get a little crispy.

This works well as a side dish or even as a snack. It's even good cold!

## VARIATIONS:

The flavor combinations are endless, have fun with it!

## Build-Your-Own Trail Mix
Makes 1 quart

### INGREDIENTS
½ cup whole nuts
½ cup whole nuts
½ cup dried fruit
½ cup dried fruit
¼-½ cup specialty ingredient
Optional: ½ cup seeds
Optional: ¼-½ tsp. spice

### DIRECTIONS:
- Mix all items together until combined.
- Store in airtight jar in cool cupboard.

### VARIATIONS:
1. Raw almonds, macadamia nuts, dried cranberries, dried pineapple, raw pumpkin seeds, and shredded coconut
2. Raw or roasted almonds, walnuts, dried cranberries, raisins, sunflower seeds, and mini chocolate chips (optional ¼ tsp. cinnamon)
3. Raw cashews, walnuts, dried blueberries, dried cherries, pumpkin seeds and yogurt covered raisins.
4. Raw almond, raw cashews, dried coconut pcs., dried mango pcs., ¼ tsp. cayenne pepper(spicy!)

The possibilities are endless and there are tons of great recipes online if you'd like some more inspiration.

## Side Dish Recipes

### <u>Gluten-Free Fried Rice</u>
Serves 8

### INGREDIENTS:
3 strips bacon, diced
1 carrot, finely chopped
¼ onion, finely chopped
3 ribs celery, finely chopped
3 cups cooked brown rice
Tamari - gluten-free soy sauce
Handful of chives or 2 green onions, sliced

### DIRECTIONS:
- Cook bacon in large skillet until browned.
- Add onion, celery and carrots and cook until soft, about 8 mins.
- Add rice and stir until combined.
- Add gluten-free soy sauce little by little and mix as you go until just tan in color.
- Top with chives and serve warm.

### VARIATIONS:
1. Add steamed broccoli or frozen peas with the veggies.
2. Skip the bacon and fry an egg instead. Break the yolk and cook egg in a patty shape. Once cooked through slice into ¼" strips and set aside. Add back in with

soy sauce.

3. Add any leftover diced meat for added variety--steak, chicken, pork loin or chops.

## Quasi Risotto

Serves 4

### INGREDIENTS:

1 small onion, diced

8 thin asparagus spears, cut into 1" pcs. (woody ends removed)

1 zucchini, quartered lengthwise and cut into ¼" pcs.

2 garlic cloves, minced

1 cup chicken or vegetable broth

1 cup frozen peas, thawed

3 cups cooked rice (any rice works, arborio is traditional for risotto and will result in a creamier dish)

2 green onions, cut into ¼" pcs.

3 Tbs. butter

¾ cup parmesan cheese, grated

1-2 Tbs. fresh basil, sliced (or ½ tsp. dried)

Salt and pepper to taste

### DIRECTIONS:

- In a large skillet, cover and sauté onion, asparagus and zucchini in 2 Tbs. olive oil until bright green and beginning to soften, about 4 mins on medium heat.
- Stir in garlic until fragrant, about 30 seconds.
- Add chicken stock, peas, green onions, rice, and butter mix to combine.
- Cook over medium heat for 2 minutes.
- Add parmesan cheese and basil, stir to combine.
- Remove from heat and add salt and pepper to taste.
- Serve warm.

# Quinoa Pesto Three Bean Salad

Serves 8

This recipe calls for canned beans. Are canned beans the best option? Well, no. But this recipe is great to have in your back pocket for those busy weeks when you just need something quick!

## INGREDIENTS:

1 can green beans
1 can cannellini beans
1 can kidney beans
4 oz. pesto sauce
Optional: 1 cup cooked quinoa

## DIRECTIONS:

- Open cans of beans.
- Drain and rinse beans.
- Add all beans, pesto and quinoa (if desired) to a large bowl.
- Mix gently until combined.

This recipe is a great side dish, potluck dish or it even works as an easy packed lunch.

Oh, and did you know quinoa can be cooked in your rice cooker just as easily as rice?!

# Gluten-Free Minestrone

Serves 8

## INGREDIENTS:

1 yellow onion, diced

3 celery stalks, diced

3 carrots, diced

2 zucchini, quartered lengthwise and sliced into ¼" pcs.

½ cup red wine (optional)

6 cups chicken or vegetable broth

1 can diced tomatoes with juice

1 bunch swiss chard, chopped

1 cup small gluten-free pasta

½ tsp. dried oregano

½ tsp. dried parsley

1 Tbs. fresh basil (or 1 tsp. dried basil)

Parmesan cheese for topping

## DIRECTIONS:

- In a large soup pot over medium heat, sauté onion, celery, carrots and zucchini in 2 Tbs. olive oil until just beginning to soften, about 2 minutes.
- Add red wine and continue to cook until wine is reduced to about ¼ cup, 4 minutes.
- Add broth, tomatoes with juice, and swiss chard.
- Cover and bring to a slow boil.
- Cook covered for about 10 minutes.
- Add pasta and continue slow boil until pasta is done, about 8 minutes.

- Reduce heat to low.
- Add oregano, parsley and basil, if using dried basil.
- Stir to combine and allow to simmer on low for an additional 5-10 minutes.
- Salt and pepper to taste.
- Serve warm and top with parmesan cheese and fresh basil.

# Sausage Stuffed Zucchini

Serves 6

## INGREDIENTS:

4 medium zucchini

½ yellow onion, diced finely

2 cloves garlic, minced

1 rib celery, diced finely

4 sweet Italian sausages, peeled

¼ cup dry white wine (or chicken broth)

3 Tbs. fresh basil, chopped (or 2 tsp. dried basil)

1 tsp. fresh rosemary, chopped

½ tsp. salt

½ tsp. pepper

2 Tbs. butter

¾ cup gluten-free Italian breadcrumbs

1 egg, beaten

## DIRECTIONS:

- Preheat oven to 375°F.
- Remove zucchini stem and cut in half lengthwise.
- Use a spoon to scoop only the soft center flesh of the zucchini.
- Reserve and dice the insides and set aside.
- In a skillet on medium heat, sauté onions and celery in 1 Tbs. olive oil until beginning to soften, about 4 mins.
- Add zucchini insides and garlic.
- Cook an additional 2 minutes.

- Add wine or broth and cook down for about 2 minutes.
- Add sausage meat, break apart and cook until brown.
- Add basil, rosemary, salt, pepper and butter.
- Mix to combine and cook additional 2 minutes.
- Remove from heat and allow to cool in a large mixing bowl.
- Once meat is cool add egg and breadcrumbs.
- Mix completely.
- Fill zucchini shells to heaping.
- Fill 9" x 13" baking dish with ¼"- ½" water.
- Place filled zucchini's in the pan.
- Bake until golden brown and zucchini is soft all the way through when poked with a fork, about 25-45 mins. depending on the size of the zucchini.
- Serve warm with grated parmesan

## Main Dish Recipes

### <u>Gluten-Free Quiche</u>

Serves 8

**INGREDIENTS:**

1 pie crust, ready for filling

½ yellow onion, chopped

1 red bell pepper, diced

1 small zucchini, quartered lengthwise and sliced

1-2 garlic cloves, minced

2 cups fresh spinach, rough chopped

4 eggs

3 Tbs. gluten-free all-purpose flour blend

½ tsp. baking powder

1 cup coconut milk (whole milk works too)

½ tsp. salt

¼ tsp. pepper

½ tsp. dried oregano

½ tsp. dried parsley (or a handful of fresh, chopped)

**DIRECTIONS:**

- Preheat oven to 350°F.
- In a skillet on medium heat, sauté onion, bell pepper, zucchini with 1 Tbs. olive oil until soft, about 6 minutes, stirring frequently.
- Add garlic and spinach, mix to combine.
- Add scant ¼ cup water and cover.
- Continue to cook for 2 minutes until spinach is soft.

- Remove cover and cook off any excess water.
- Remove from heat.
- In a large mixing bowl beat eggs well.
- Add milk, spices, baking powder and flour, mix until combined.
- Add veggies to egg mixture and mix until combined.
- Transfer mixture to prepared pie crust.
- Bake until eggs are set, about 45-50 minutes.
- Begin checking on quiche at about 35 minutes--if the crust starts to get too brown, use aluminum foil to cover only the crust so it does not burn.

## VARIATIONS:

1. Quasi Quiche:
   No time for a crust, no problem. Mix ½ cup dried quinoa in the mixture and omit the flour. The quinoa will fall to the bottom forming a quasi crust!

2. Spinach and Cream Cheese
   Mix 3 oz. of cream cheese well with the eggs in the first step and reduce the milk to ½ cup. Replace the zucchini with an additional cup of fresh spinach.

## Gluten-Free Salmon Cakes
Serves 4

### INGREDIENTS:
2 cans boneless skinless salmon, drained
2 eggs
½ lemon, zest and juice
1 tsp. Dried dill
Handful of chives, finely chopped
¾ cup plain gluten-free breadcrumbs

### DIRECTIONS:
- Add salmon and everything except ½ cup breadcrumbs to large bowl and mix to combine.
- Make into 4 patties and refrigerate for 10 mins to set.
- Heat skillet with 3 Tbs. olive oil on medium heat.
- Coat patties in breadcrumbs and place in pan.
- Cook, turning once until golden brown, about 8 minutes.

These keep well for lunch the next day. Add to the top of a salad for an easy no-heat meal!

## Burrito Bowls
Serves 4

### INGREDIENTS:
3 cups lettuce, shredded
2 cups cooked brown rice
1 lb. cooked ground beef
1 can black beans, drained and rinsed
2 tomatoes, diced
Optional: shredded cheese
Optional: guacamole or diced avocados
Optional: sour cream
Optional: salsa

### DIRECTIONS:
- In individual bowls layer all ingredients in order OR make it a build-your-own night and let everyone build it themselves!

### VARIATIONS:
1. Replace beef with chicken.
2. Add corn.
3. Top with broken corn tortilla chips from the bottom of the bag.
4. Add sautéed sliced onions and bell peppers.

This one is so easy--mix it up!

# Italian Stuffed Bell Peppers

Serves 8

## INGREDIENTS:

4 green bell peppers, seeded and halved
2 cups cooked brown rice
½ yellow onion, diced
2 cloves garlic, minced
1 lb. ground beef
1 small can diced tomatoes, drained (or tomato purée)
½ tsp. dried basil
½ tsp. dried oregano
¼ tsp. salt
¼ tsp. pepper
1 egg, beaten
¾ cup parmesan cheese, grated

## DIRECTIONS:

- Preheat oven to 350°F.
- In a skillet over medium heat sauté onion until soft, about 4 minutes.
- Add garlic and stir until fragrant, about 1 minute.
- Add ground beef breaking it apart and cook until brown.
- Drain fat from the pan.
- Transfer to a mixing bowl and allow to cool.
- Add tomatoes, spices, egg, cheese and mix to combine.
- Stuff peppers.

- Fill 9" x 13" baking dish with ½" water and set filled peppers in the dish.
- Cover with foil and bake until pepper is cooked through and soft, about 35-45 mins.

## VARIATIONS:

1. Use artichokes instead! Place stuffing between the leaves of trimmed artichoke and increase baking time to 1½ hours.

# Cheeseburger Pizza

Makes 1 pizza

## INGREDIENTS:

1 pizza crust, ready for toppings
6-8 strips nitrate-free bacon, diced
1 tomato, sliced
1 cup mozzarella, shredded
1 Tbs. mayonnaise
1 Tbs. ketchup
2 tsp. of dill pickle relish
2 cups lettuce, shredded

## DIRECTIONS:

- Preheat oven as per directions for the crust.
- In a pan cook bacon over medium heat until cooked through and crispy.
- Save 1 Tbs. of bacon grease and set aside.
- Strain bacon and place on a paper towel lined plate.
- Mix mayonnaise, ketchup and pickle relish in a small mixing bowl until combined.
- Using a brush spread reserved bacon grease to the pizza crust.
- Evenly distribute the cooked bacon on the crust.
- Place tomatoes on crust.
- Top with cheese. It will look sparse, that is okay.
- Bake pizza in oven for 8-10 minutes until cheese is just melted and crust looks done.
- While pizza is baking toss the lettuce with the

ketchup mixture until evenly coated.
- When pizza is done allow to cool for 5 minutes.
- Add lettuce topping.
- Slice and serve.

# Kid-Friendly Pesto Pasta

Serves 4

## INGREDIENTS:

12 oz. of gluten-free spaghetti or pasta of your choice

## Sauce:

4 handfuls of spinach leaves (about 3 cups)
1 handful of Italian parsley leaves (about 1 cup)
¼ cup whole raw walnuts
½ cup grated parmesan cheese
2 cloves garlic, minced
1 Tbs. lemon juice
Good pinch of salt
½ cup olive oil

## DIRECTIONS:

- Cook pasta as directed.
- While the pasta is cooking make the sauce.
- Add spinach, parsley, walnuts, parmesan, lemon juice and garlic to the food processor.
- Pulse until well combined and nuts are broken down.
- Scrape down sides if necessary.
- Through the top add olive oil while the processor is running.
- Add more oil if the pesto looks too much like a paste. It should be a bit oily.
- Add salt to taste.

- Once the pasta is drained mix the pesto with the pasta.
- If you have any leftover pesto it will keep in an airtight container in the fridge for a week.

## VARIATION:

You can absolutely use basil for part or all of the greens. I have found that most children are much more receptive to the milder spinach and parsley flavors over that of basil.

# 30-Minute Veggie Chili
Serves 6

## INGREDIENTS:
1 can black beans, drained and rinsed
3 medium zucchini, diced
1 small to medium onion, diced
1 cup frozen corn, thawed
4 cloves garlic, minced
1 Tbs. chili powder
1 Tbs. cumin
¼ tsp. cayenne
2 cups vegetable broth
1 can diced fire-roasted tomatoes
1 lime, juiced
Optional: 1 jalapeño, seeded and diced finely

## DIRECTIONS:
- Cook zucchini and onion over medium heat with 2 Tbs. of olive oil until soft, about 5 mins.
- Add corn, garlic and spices. Mix until combined, about 1 minute.
- Stir in broth, tomatoes with juice and jalapeños, if using.
- Mash the beans a bit with a fork.
- Add beans to the pot.
- Cover and simmer for 15 minutes.
- Uncover and continue to simmer until desired thickness.

- Remove from heat and stir in lime juice.

Serve topped with cheese, avocado, diced tomatoes and onions, or hot sauce. And don't forget the gluten-free tortillas!

# Gluten-Free "Fried" Chicken

Serves 8

## INGREDIENTS:

4 skinless bone-in chicken breasts

4 skinless bone-in chicken thighs

3 cups cashew milk (regular milk works as well)

3 Tbs. white vinegar

5 cloves garlic, minced

2 cups gluten-free Italian breadcrumbs

½ cup parmesan cheese, grated

1 tsp. salt

1½ tsp. pepper

## DIRECTIONS:

- Mix milk and vinegar and set aside 5 minutes.
- Add garlic to milk mixture.
- Soak chicken in milk mixture in refrigerator for at least 30 mins (up to 10 hours).
- Preheat oven to 425°F.
- Mix breadcrumbs, salt, pepper and parmesan cheese in a wide flat bowl or pie plate for dredging.
- Coat in breadcrumbs.
- Let stand on parchment paper or wire rack for 15 minutes.
- Coat again in breadcrumbs.
- Place on parchment lined cookie sheet and drizzle lightly with olive oil.
- Bake for 45-50 mins until crisp and internal temperature is 165°F.

# Gluten-Free Mini Meatloaf
Serves 6

## INGREDIENTS:
1½ lb. ground beef
1 cup mushrooms, finely chopped
1 small onion, finely chopped
¾ cup gluten-free bread crumbs
12 oz. can tomato sauce
2 eggs
¼ cup parsley, chopped (or 1 Tbs. dried)
½ tsp. sea salt
¼ tsp. pepper
¼ tsp. crushed red pepper

## Sauce:
3 tsp. apple cider vinegar
3 Tbs. brown sugar

## DIRECTIONS:
- Preheat oven to 450°F.
- Mix all ingredients except ½ of the tomato sauce, until just combined.
- Do not overmix.
- Shape into 6 even mini-loafs.
- Heat skillet over medium heat with 1 Tbs. oil.
- When skillet is warm add loaves.
- Cook until each side is brown, taking care when turning.

- Meanwhile, mix remaining tomato sauce with 1 tsp. brown sugar and 1 Tbs. apple cider vinegar.
- Once all sides are brown, add sauce to top of each loaf.
- Place skillet in oven for 20-25 mins or until internal temperature of largest loaf is 165°F.

## Special Treat Recipes

### Chocolate Peanut Butter Crispy Rice Delight
Makes 18 squares

### INGREDIENTS:
6 cups crispy rice cereal
4 dates, pitted
1 cup smooth peanut butter (or nut butter of your choice)
½ cup maple syrup

### Topping:
12 oz. chocolate chips
½ cup peanut butter (or nut butter of your choice)
1 tsp. coconut oil

### DIRECTIONS:
- Grease a 9" x 13" baking dish.
- Add crispy rice cereal to a large mixing bowl.
- Run dates, peanut butter, honey and maple through food processor until mixture sticks together.
- Add mixture to rice cereal and use your hands to incorporate until all cereal is combined.
- Press mixture firmly into prepared baking dish.
- In the small pot or double boiler add the additional peanut butter, chocolate chips and coconut oil.
- Warm slowly, stirring constantly until melted.
- Pour chocolate mixture over cereal in the baking dish.

- Spread the chocolate topping with a spatula or knife to smooth it out.
- Allow to cool in fridge until chocolate is hard, about 1 hour.
- Cut into squares as you serve.

# Gluten-Free Oatmeal Chocolate Chip Cookies
Makes 24 cookies

## INGREDIENTS:
2 cups gluten-free all-purpose flour blend
2½ cups gluten-free rolled oats
1 tsp. baking powder
¼ tsp. salt
10 Tbs. unsalted butter, melted and cooled
¾ cup sugar
1 cup brown sugar
2 eggs
½ tsp. vanilla extract
¼ cup cashew milk (regular milk works too)
12 oz. chocolate chips

## DIRECTIONS:
- Preheat oven to 375°F.
- In a large mixing bowl combine flour, oats, baking powder and salt.
- In a separate bowl combine butter, sugar and brown sugar.
- Add eggs, vanilla and milk. Mix well.
- Add wet ingredients to dry and mix until combined.
- Add chocolate chips and mix until combined.
- Spoon batter in ~¼ cup scoops onto ungreased cookie sheet, leaving about 2" in between.

- Bake on middle shelf for 12-15 minutes, until cookies are beginning to turn golden brown at bottom edges.
- Transfer cookies to wire rack to cool.

# Gluten-Free Apple Crumble
Serves 6

## INGREDIENTS:
4-5 apples, peeled, cored and diced (a mix of Gala and Granny Smith works best)
1 Tbs. sugar
1 tsp. cinnamon
¼ tsp. nutmeg
2 cup gluten-free rolled oats
½ cup gluten-free all-purpose flour blend
⅓ cup coconut or date sugar (brown sugar also works)
8 Tbs. butter, cubed

## DIRECTIONS:
- Preheat oven to 350°F.
- Grease 9" x 9" baking dish.
- Mix apples cinnamon, nutmeg and sugar until apples are coated.
- Transfer apples to baking dish.
- Mix oats, flour and 4 Tbs. of the butter in a mixing bowl, cutting through the butter until all pieces are broken up.
- Add coconut sugar and mix until combined.
- Top apples with flour mixture.
- Dot top of mixture with remaining butter.
- Bake for 30 minutes until bubbly and topping is beginning to brown.
- Serve warm with or without vanilla ice cream.

# CHAPTER 10

## RESOURCE GUIDE

# Information and Tips on Gluten-Free Living

Explanations, Tips & Advice:
- www.glutenfreegluten.com
- www.foodallergy.org/allergens/wheat-allergy
- www.glutenintoleranceschool.com
- www.glutenfreehelp.info
- www.celiac.org/live-gluten-free/glutenfreediet/

Complete List of Grains & Flours and Their Gluten Content:
- www.csaceliacs.org/grains_and_flours_glossary.jsp

Where to Turn for Gluten-Free Restaurants:
This app gives a listing of restaurants with gluten-free menu options. There is also a filter that you can use to find dedicated gluten-free facilities and those with dedicated gluten-free fryers.

App and Website: www.findmeglutenfree.com/

List of Gluten-Free Foods From Around The World:
This website lists dishes from all different types of cuisines that are traditionally gluten free.

www.gluten-free-around-the-world.com/

## Shopping List App

Wunderlist App - www.wunderlist.com

## Recommended Gluten-Free Products

Best Gluten-Free Bread Flour Mix
- Pamela's® Gluten-Free Bread Mix
- King Arthur® Gluten-Free Bread Mix

Recommended Gluten-Free All-Purpose Flour Blends
- Pamela's® All Purpose Flour - Artisan Blend
- Better Batter® Gluten-Free Flour
- King Arthur® Gluten-Free Measure for Measure Flour
- Bob's Red Mill® Gluten-Free 1:1 Baking Flour

Best Gluten-Free Breads
- Canyon Bakehouse® - Sandwich bread, cinnamon raisin, hamburger buns and bagels
- Schar® - Baguettes and ciabatta
- Three Bakers® - Hot dog buns
- Rudi's Organic Bakery® - Sandwich bread

Gluten-Free Pizza Crust
- Pamela's® or King Arthur Bread Mix - Make your own
- Udi's® - Pre-made frozen pizza crust
- Three Bakers® - Pre-made pizza crust

Gluten-Free Pie Crust
-   Pillsbury® - Pre-made pie crust

Gluten-Free Cake Mixes
-   Arrowhead Mills® cake mixes
-   King Arthur® cake mixes
-   Wholesome Chow® cake mixes

Gluten-Free Brownie Mix
-   Arrowhead Mills® Gluten-Free Fudge Brownie Mix

## Sources for Great Gluten-Free Recipes

Great Gluten-Free Recipe Sources
-   www.glutenfreeonashoestring.com
    -   Breads and baked goods
    -   Gluten-free replacements of all your name brand favorites
-   www.elanaspantry.com
    -   Paleo recipes, completely grain-free, and super delicious
-   www.nogluten-noproblem.com
    -   Gluten-free recipes for the whole family

Great Recipe Sources That Aren't Exclusively Gluten Free
-   www.americastestkitchen.com
    -   Fool-proof recipes of your family favorites

- www.mywholefoodlife.com
    - Refrigerator oats
    - Snack bars
    - Breakfast cookies
    - Sweet treats
- www.minimalistbaker.com
    - Delicious recipes with 10 ingredients or less

## Interesting Information

Information on Celiac Disease And Gluten Intolerance
- www.nlm.nih.gov/medlineplus/celiacdisease.html
- www.Celiac.org
- www.BeyondCeliac.org
- www.glutenintoleranceschool.com

Research on Gluten
- https://www.ncbi.nlm.nih.gov/pubmed/

Research on Gut Bacteria
- www.ted.com/talks/rob_knight_how_our_microbes_make_us_who_we_are

# References

1.  Glyphosate as a Pre-harvest Aid in Small Grains. (2014, July, 7). North Dakota State University. Retrieved from https://www.ag.ndsu.edu/cpr/plant-science/glyphosate-as-a-pre-harvest-aid-in-small-grains-07-17-14

2.  Preharvest Staging Guide. (2012, August, 10). Monsanto. Retrieved from http://roundup.ca/_uploads/documents/MON-Preharvest%20Staging%20Guide.pdf

3.  Roseboro, Ken. (2016, February, 25). Grim reaping: Many food crops sprayed with weed killer before harvest. The Organic and Non-GMO Report. Retrieved from http://non-gmoreport.com/articles/grim-reaper-many-food-crops-sprayed-with-weed-killer-before-harvest/

4.  O'Brien, Robyn. (2010). Allergy Kids Foundation. Retrieved from https://robynobrien.com/allergy-kids-foundation/

5.  GMO Science For The Beginner. (2015-2016). GMO Science. Retrieved from https://www.gmoscience.org/for-the-beginner/

6.  Questions and Answers: Gluten-Free Food Labeling Final Rule. (2016, May, 2). United States Food and Drug Administration. Retrieved from

http://www.fda.gov/Food/GuidanceRegulation/
GuidanceDocumentsRegulatoryInformation/Allergens/
ucm362880.htm

7.  Gluten and Food Labeling. (2016, May, 2). United States
Food and Drug Administration. Retrieved from http://www.
fda.gov/Food/ResourcesForYou/Consumers/ucm367654.
htm

8.  Kasim S. et al. (2007). Nonresponsive Celiac Disease
Due to Inhaled Gluten. New England Journal of Medicine.
Retrieved from
https://www.verywell.com/suffering-symptoms-from-
airborne-gluten-562332

9. Duke SO, Powles SB. (2008). Glyphosate: a once-in-a-century
herbicide. Pest Management Science.  64:319 – 325 (2008).
Retrieved from http://naldc.nal.usda.gov/download/17918/
PDF

10.  Vrain Dr., Thierry. (2014, October, 27).  A letter to the
Minister of Health. Retrieved from https://robynobrien.com/
a-former-gmo-scientist-sends-an-open-letter-to-canadas-
minister-of-health/

THE ESSENTIAL GLUTEN-FREE GUIDE

# Appendix A
Gluten Diseases, Intolerances and Sensitivities Explained

<u>Celiac Disease</u>
We know that as many as 1.8 million people in the United States suffer from celiac disease and cannot tolerate gluten. Celiac disease is an autoimmune condition which is different from an allergy. In people with celiac disease, as in anyone with autoimmune disease, the immune system that is meant to protect the body from invaders, like viruses and foreign bacteria, begins attacking the body's own cells.

When a person with celiac disease eats something that contains even the smallest amount of gluten it triggers his or her body to attack the lining, or the villi, of the small intestine. The intestinal villi are key players in the nutrient absorption for the body. This can be detrimental to the health of the patient. Symptoms of celiac disease can vary from intestinal problems (like bloating, diarrhea and abdominal cramps) to issues related to malnutrition (such as joint pain, weight loss, vitamin and mineral deficiencies, skin rashes and chronic fatigue).

How can you tell if you have celiac disease? There are a series of blood tests that can detect elevated levels of antibodies which give your doctor a good idea of what is going on in your body. However negative blood tests don't necessarily mean that you don't have celiac and blood tests can yield false positives as well. For this reason, blood tests are often followed by an endoscopy so your doctor can take a look at your small intestine to make a final determination on the diagnosis and the extent of damage to the intestinal wall. Also, it is important to note that for accurate testing you must be on a gluten-containing diet.

For more information on celiac disease visit: www.nlm.nih. gov/medlineplus/celiacdisease.html

Wheat Allergy
A wheat allergy is distinctly different from celiac disease and its symptoms are just that--an allergic reaction, or an over-reaction of the immune system to a specific trigger, in this case wheat. In an allergic reaction, the immune system does not attack the person's own cells, as it does with an autoimmune disease, but it is no less potentially harmful. Symptoms of a wheat allergy can result in a variety of reactions ranging from a rash and itching to swelling or even difficulty breathing or loss of consciousness. Food allergies like this can be immediately life threatening and should not be taken lightly. Strict avoidance of all wheat products is required. Wheat allergy (as with most food allergies) can be diagnosed with a simple blood test or skin prick test.

For more information on wheat allergy visit: www.foodallergy. org/allergens/wheat-allergy

## Non-Celiac Gluten Sensitivity

Non-celiac gluten sensitivity or (NCGS) encompasses a wide variety of symptoms exhibited in patients that do not have celiac disease or a wheat allergy and whose symptoms are significantly reduced or disappear completely with adherence to a gluten-free diet. Symptoms can vary from intestinal issues that mirror those of celiac or irritable bowel syndrome (IBS) to a host of other non-intestinal symptoms ranging from mental fogginess and some psychiatric issues to skin rashes, joint pain and some autoimmune disorders such as Hashimoto's--all of which improve with the implementation of a gluten-free diet.

NCGS is a newly recognized medical condition within the medical community. It was first discovered in the 1980's however it was as recently as 2011 when results were published by two well-respected celiac physicians that people began to look at it more closely. Still today, though, many doctors don't take the condition seriously. Because specific biomarkers have yet to be identified and no proven diagnostic test, NCGS remains controversial.

## Gluten Intolerance

Gluten intolerance is another term you hear thrown around. It is not a specific ailment, but instead is an umbrella term that covers all forms of gluten issues including, but not limited to: celiac disease, wheat allergy, and NCGS.

## Dermatitis Herpetiformis

This term refers to a type of gluten sensitivity resulting in a specific type of rash. It can be found in conjunction with celiac, on its own or possibly in conjunction with NCGS. It is characterized by a group of small blisters that is extremely itchy. It is relatively rare and diagnosed by a skin biopsy. Strict adherence to a gluten-free diet is strongly recommended to manage this agonizing condition.

## Gluten Ataxia

Gluten ataxia is also very rare and still a bit of a mystery for the medical community. It is believed that in gluten ataxia, gluten triggers an immune response that results in decreased voluntary muscle control. Though the mechanism is not completely understood, it is possible that the loss of motor control is the result of excess antibodies being deposited in the part of the brain responsible for motor skills. In short, it is another example that points to a glitch in the immune response triggered by gluten.

For more information on Non-Celiac gluten intolerances visit: www.glutenintoleranceschool.com

# Appendix B
### Round-up® In Your Body

You may find it interesting that every article I could find defending or denying the practice of using Round-up® to speed up the drying process of wheat just prior to harvest was written by someone who is in some way associated with Monsanto, the company that manufactures Round-up®.

It is also noteworthy that the main ingredient in Round-up®, glyphosate, is listed as a probable carcinogen by the World Health Organization. Furthermore, the mechanism used in glyphosate for killing weeds is one that disrupts the Shikimate Pathway, a pathway that allows for the biosynthesis of three very important amino acids.[9] This pathway is only found in plants and microorganisms.

As it happens, the gut bacteria of humans also depend on the shikimate pathway.[10] Have you noticed that we are also all of a sudden talking a whole lot about probiotics? Could Round-up® be killing off our gut bacteria and leaving us sick?

Our gut bacteria or flora are extremely important to our health. It is said that 70% of our immune system is located in the gut. If you are at all interested in this there is a TED Talk that does a great job of explaining the basics. Take a look--it's quite fascinating:

www.ted.com/talks/rob_knight_how_our_microbes_make_us_who_we_are

# Appendix C
Bonus Material

To make sure you have everything you need at your fingertips, I have made all of the resources in this book available to you with clickable links and in printable formats at:

www.healthyana.net/essentialgf

At this link you will find:
- Printable cheat sheet for flours and grains that are aligned with a gluten-free diet.
- Printable cheat sheet of ingredients that contain hidden gluten.
- List of all recommended products.
- List of all recommended recipe sources with clickable links.
- Printable versions of all recipes included in the book.
- Printable cheat sheet for gluten-free substitutions.
- Printable cheat sheet for gluten-free baking.

Plus, I will continue to collect and share great gluten-free recipes!

Go to: www.healthyana.net/essentialgf

And get started, today!

Made in the USA
Middletown, DE
21 December 2016